KETO DIET COOKBOOK FOR WOMEN OVER 50

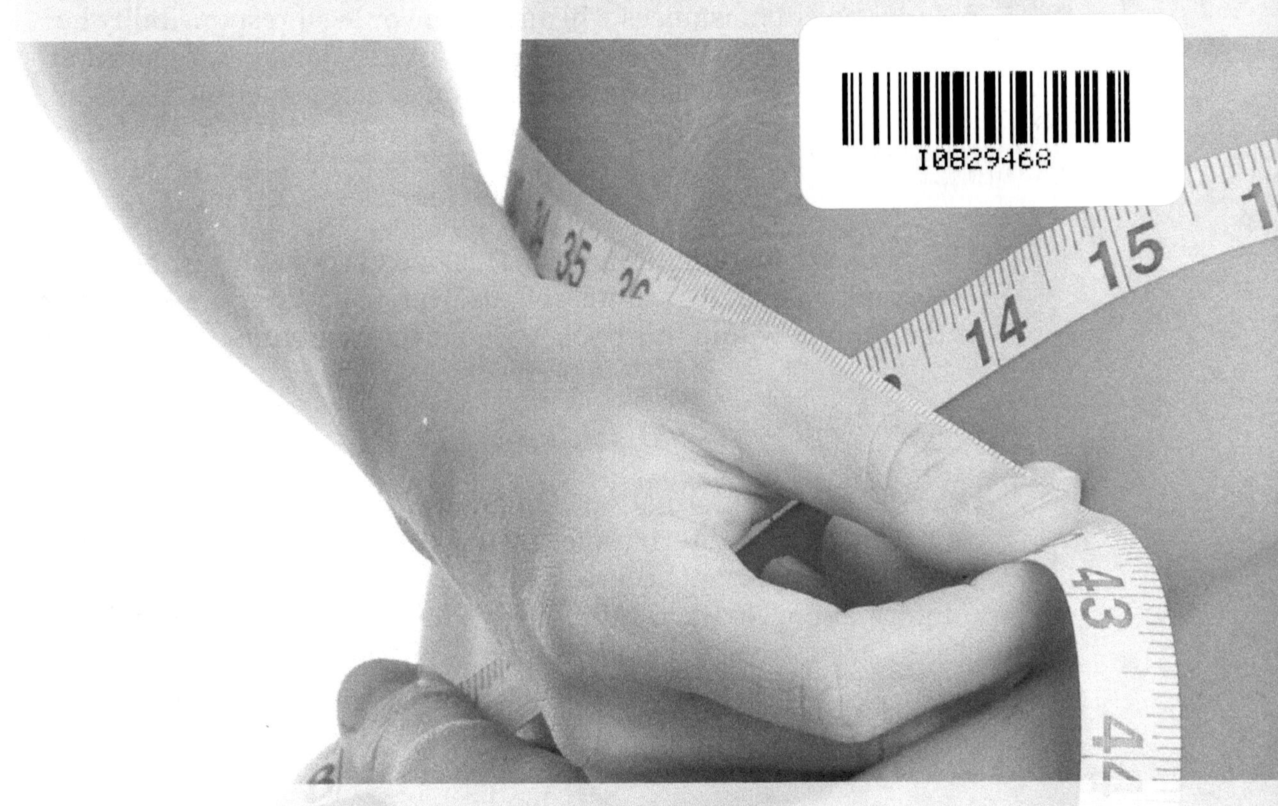

The Proven and Ultimate Weight Loss Diet Program to Boost Your Weight Loss Fast and Easy for a Healthy Lifestyle Metabolism Management

STEPHANIE ROBBINS

TABLE OF CONTENTS

INTRODUCTION

Keto diet is a combination of high fat and low carb. The diet has been helpful for so many people in achieving great weight loss results. It is not just a weight loss diet, but it helps us to be healthy.

Ar first, the keto diet is very simple. It is a diet where the person is required to stop eating foods that contain lots of carbs (sugar) and start eating foods that have high-fat content. Keto diet is mostly associated with high protein intake. While people are aware that it is possible to achieve weight loss through the keto diet only, the majority of them are not aware that it is possible to build muscles with the help of keto. Getting your muscles in shape is fun with keto. It does not matter if you are male or female you can achieve what you want with keto.

For women over 50 years of age, a keto diet is one of the best diets. With keto, they will lose their anxiety over food, and never again they will have to worry about calories. The diet is very easy to follow. There is nothing to follow. You are free to eat anything which you want as long as it is not carb. It is also necessary to maintain the ratio of fat/protein and carbohydrates so you can achieve your goals of weight loss or muscle gaining according to your desire. Because of the changes occurring in the bodies of women over 50, it is imperative to look at how the needs of these women are different from younger women and men. During menopause, hormones shift in women, and these changes make it necessary to make some adjustments to their lifestyle in general, and diet in particular.

General Nutritional Needs for Women Over 50

Bone density decreases, making it necessary to increase the amount of vitamin D and calcium consumed in order to maintain adequate bone density as the body ages. All this, combined with a reduction in the number of calories needed to fuel the body, makes it necessary to modify the diet as a woman enters postmenopausal years. These natural changes to the body make changes to the diet necessary as a woman ages.

Also, as women age, their ability to discern thirstiness may diminish. Water consumption is still an important factor in the health of a woman. Because it is harder to determine thirst as you surpass your 50th year, it is essential that you consume 8 to 9 8-oz. glasses of water each day. Drink more in the winter, in hot weather and when exercising. While you are drinking more water, it may serve to curb your appetite. This is good because you will need to lower your caloric intake from what you may be used to. This happens when you are finding new aches and pains and slowing down your exercise regime. Exercise may be less intense as you make modifications to coincide with your age and decreases in mobility. This is because you are not as flexible and may be experiencing inflammation in your joints. While these are all relatively normal signs of aging, the decrease in physical activity may cause additional problems in the form of weight gain.

This may be a good time to eliminate processed foods and sugar from your diet. Dietary fiber is the key to avoiding constipation. Studies show that women over 50 may be up to seven times more likely to suffer from constipation than men of a similar age. Failure on consuming enough dietary fiber can result in small, hard stool. It is beneficial to consume dietary fiber, which is found in whole grains, and food that is made from whole grains, as well as fruits and vegetables. The foods move through the intestines easily and make solid stool that moves through the intestines quickly and efficiently. The dietary fiber in these foods may help in lowering bad cholesterol (LDL) levels in adults. This may have a positive effect on heart health as well. Since estrogen levels in women are also decreasing, the female body begins to lose the positive effect estrogen has on the heart and blood vessels. This is another impact of menopause. Consuming adequate amounts of dietary fiber may help to improve heart health.

Gentler Approach to Keto for Women Over 50

Women over 50 may want to modify their keto approach by increasing the daily carbohydrates to 100 to 150 g per day. They may also want to increase the protein from 25% to 30% of the diet. The remaining amount of food will be fat. The increased carbohydrates provide less distress to hormones and metabolism and put less stress on the body while adjusting to a diet low in carbohydrates. The increase in protein is to offset the body's tendency to lose muscle mass as women age. Additionally, the carbs will provide energy to exercise. The metabolisms of women typically slow as women age. The increase in carbs and protein may allow women over 50 to forgo the sluggish feelings and allow enough energy to exercise while on the diet. This will improve overall health. Carbohydrates in your diet should come from whole grains or high-quality carbs like pumpkins, carrots, spaghetti squash, and small quantities of butternut squash. Foods that grow below the ground have higher carbohydrate content. If you feel like you need to sneak them into your diet, it should be small amounts per serving. They add variety and flavor to your diet, but they must be used in moderation. Even with a few extra carbs in your diet, you should be able to enter ketosis. The same is true for protein. The body may not enter ketosis as quickly, but the effects of the changes will not be as hostile to your body and the immune system.

The keto diet sets the importance of high-fiber low-carb food. Be sure to include leafy greens and healthy oils in your diet. The leafy greens will help avoid gastrointestinal issues during keto. They contain the fiber lost with the reduction of carbohydrates. Many vegetables contain carbohydrates, so be aware of the amount you are eating and stay within your macros. Some of the vegetables have fiber and no carbohydrates, but others, like cauliflower and jicama, have carbs. You must remember to count them in your daily totals. Green leafy vegetables have protein that must be added as well. Overall, it is best to get your fiber from vegetables to keep you energized and lessen the effects of keto flu and keto diarrhea, as well as constipation.

1. MENOPAUSE

The keto diet has become very popular in recent years because of the success people have noticed. There's a lot that the ketogenic diet does to help you reach a healthy and balanced weight and stay there: restore insulin sensitivity levels, build and maintain muscle mass, and lower inflammation. A woman who consumes way too many carbohydrates can jump-start menopause signs. Let's have a look at how a ketogenic diet can aid with the signs and symptoms of menopause.

Way # 1 - Controlling Insulin Levels

By going on a ketogenic diet, women with PCOS (polycystic ovary syndrome) can help regulate their hormones. The researchers studied the effect of low-glycemic diets have shown this impact. PCOS triggers insulin sensitivity concerns, to be helped by insulin-reducing properties of low-glycemic carbohydrates.

Way # 2 - You'll Have More Energy

Our bodies will experience widely known energy dips if we fuel them with mainly sugar and carbohydrates. Especially if you take in quick and refined sugars (think about carrot cake, cupcakes, crackers, bread, candy, etc.) Changes in blood glucose can stop by receiving a steady amount of sugar. High blood glucose makes the body send insulin to the pancreas, which then takes care of how muscular tissue and fat cells absorb sugar.
The reaction to the carbs consumption is a powerful release of insulin to make sure that the body can properly manage the transport of the extra sugar. With blood sugar levels down, the body will signal that it requires more sugar. This means you'll experience many energy highs and lows in one day. This can cause low energy level.

Way # 3 - Fat Burning

Menopause can trigger the metabolic process to change and reduce. One of the most common complaints of menopause is an increase in body weight and abdominal fat. A lower level of estrogen typically causes weight gain. A diet with little or no carbohydrates is very efficient for decreasing body fat. Ketosis reduces appetite by controlling the production of the "cravings hormonal agent" called ghrelin. You are less hungry while in ketosis.

Way # 4 - Reduction in Hot Flashes

Nobody totally understands hot flashes and why they take place. Hormonal changes that impact the hypothalamus, most likely have something to do with this. The hypothalamus manages the body's temperature level. Changes in hormonal agents can also disrupt this thermostat. This ends up being more sensitive to modifications in body temperature levels.
Ketones, in which its production stimulates throughout a ketogenic diet, creates a very potent source of energy for the brain. Scientists have shown that ketones act to help the hypothalamus, so the body can manage its own temperature level. The presence of ketones works to make your body's thermostat better.

Way # 5 - Excellent Night's rest

Thanks to a much steadier blood sugar level, you will improve rest while on a ketogenic diet. With even more balanced hormones and much less hot flashes, you will sleep better. Reduced stress and enhanced well-being are two of the benefits of better sleep.

2. THE KETO DIET

Although going on a keto diet offers a lot of benefits, it is important to know about what you are getting into. As a woman over her fifties, it is essential to know all the necessary to overcome challenges and achieve your long-term goal.

There will be a radical change in the way you are currently eating. The typical or standard diet is particularly high in carbohydrates, and diving into a keto diet could prove very difficult. People who adopt the ketogenic diet certainly get a series of benefits. However, before starting, you need to prepare yourself mentally, knowing, and following all the essential guidelines.
Know what to eat and avoid while on the keto diet

The meal plan for a keto diet aims to reduce carbs drastically. According to Kristen Mancinelli, a dietician based in New York and the author of The Ketogenic Diet: A Scientifically Proven Approach to Fast, Healthy Weight Loss, You can begin with an amount of 20 to 30 grams of carbohydrates every day.
You also have to know carb-rich foods, protein, and fat. This enables you to choose the foods that will keep you on a ketogenic diet wisely. You may think that only foods such as pasta, cookies, bread, ice-cream, and candy are rich in carbs. Although, for example, beans have some proteins, it is a food that is rich in carbohydrates, too. Also, many vegetables and fruits have high carbohydrate content. Foods that contain little or no carb include pure fats, butter, oils, and meat.

Know your relationship with fatty food

As a woman above 50, this is an important aspect that can't be overlooked. According to Mancinelli, the common belief of many people is that the intake of fat can kill them. Another unclear point about this is that there is currently no conclusive result in support or against this belief. According to some researches, eating polyunsaturated fats instead of saturated is essential to reduce the risk of heart disease. On the other hand, many other research studies point to the fact that total fat and various types of fats are not related to cardiovascular diseases. This controversy makes choosing what to eat a little confusing. Despite all these confusions, it is essential to note that as a woman over 50, the food you eat contains far more than one nutrient. Therefore, the important is the total quality of the diet, although more research is still needed to determine the risk and health benefits of keto.

Another factor to contemplate is that your body is not what it used to be, considering that you are now older. To prepare your body for a high-fat diet, you have to make little adjustments in your meals. For instance, you can take green vegetables instead of fries when eating burgers. You can take it up a notch and from time to time. You will begin to let your body know that a keto diet meal plan is on its way.

In situations where you should eat potatoes or rice in your meal, you can instead choose a non-starchy vegetable. When cooking, you can start using more oil, such as avocado or olive oil. You will have to do away with old dieting habits. You can't just go to make a grilled plain-looking skinless chicken breast, as this doesn't make sense when on keto. That is because it doesn't contain enough fat.
It is essential that you make up your mind on keto, as being afraid can hinder it from working. This is why it is necessary to start gradually, getting your body used to it a little at a time. Later, it will be much less complicated to push out carbs from your diet.

Foods to Eat

The Good Fats

Add Extra-Virgin Olive Oil (EVOO): Olive oil dates back centuries to a time where oil was used for anointing kings and priests.
Add Macadamia Oil: One of the benefits of this oil is its high smoke point of 390° Fahrenheit. It carries a mild flavor, which is a super alternative for olive oil in mayonnaise.

Other Monounsaturated & Saturated Fats: Include these items (listed in grams):

- Organic red palm oil, Avocado, Sesame, Olive, & Flaxseed Oil - Unsalted butter, Chicken fat, Duck fat, & Beef tallow (1 tbsp. = 0 g net carbs)
- Ghee (1 tsp. = 0 g net carbs)
- Olives (3 jumbo - 5 large/10 small = 1 g net carb)

- Unsweetened flaked coconut (2 tbsp.=3 g net carbs)

Dairy & Your Diet

Before beginning the keto way of life, you need to understand dairy and dairy products, which are an essential part of the ketogenic methods. If you're lactose intolerant, maybe the plan isn't for you. The amounts should be monitored to no more than four ounces daily. Choose dairy products that have been cultured and are keto-friendly. The number one choice is unsweetened almond milk. You can also choose from hemp milk and flax milk.

Do you know the difference between butter and ghee? Butter consists of water, milk solids, and butterfat, whereas ghee, an Indian staple, includes pure butterfat. Therefore, if you have lactose sensitivities, ghee is probably your best choice. The ghee also contains medium-chain fatty acids that assist your immune system and digestion.

Calcium

- Broccoli rabe—cooked: 3.5 ounce portion = 120 mg per 100 grams
- Greens (spinach, kale, etc.) cooked: 3.5 ounce portion = 135 mg per 100 grams
- Sesame seeds: 1 ounce portion = 273 mg per 28 grams
- Almond milk (calcium-fortified): 8 ounce portion = 300-450 mg per 225 grams
- Almonds: 1 ounce portion = 74 mg per 28 grams

Omega 3 Fatty Acids Options

Alpha-linoleic acid (ALA) is the most common omega-3 fatty acid in your diet.

The acid content is found in these using one tablespoon portions:

- Chia Seeds: 2.5 grams per 14-gram portion
- Ground Flaxseed: 1.6 grams per 7-gram portion
- Hemp Seeds: 2 grams per 20-gram portion

Iron Options

Be sure you have adequate iron in your diet. Include these food groups:

- Cooked spinach: 3.5 ounce portion = 3.6 mg per 100 grams
- Cooked white mushrooms: 3.5 ounce portion = 2.7 mg per 100 grams
- Olives: 3.5 oz. portion = 3.3 mg per 100 grams

- Sesame seeds: 1 ounce portion = 4.1 mg per 28 grams
- Pumpkin seeds: 1 ounce portion = 4.2 mg per 28 grams
- Chia seeds: 1 ounce portion = 2.2 mg per 28 grams
- Coconut milk: 3.5 oz. portion = 3.3 mg per 100 grams
- Canned hearts of palm: 3.5 oz. portion = 3.1 mg per 100 grams
- Dark chocolate: 1 ounce portion = 3.3 mg per 28 grams

Save Additional Carbohydrates

- Pasta: Replace pasta using zucchini. Use a spiralizer and make long ribbons to cover your plate. It is excellent for many dishes served this way. You can also prepare spaghetti squash for regular spaghetti.
- French Fries: Change over to zucchini fries or turnip fries.
- Tortillas: Get ready to push this one to the side, which weighs in at approximately 98 grams for one serving. Instead, enjoy a lettuce leaf at about 1 gram per serving.
- Mashed Potatoes: There's no need to prepare bowls of regular mashed potatoes; instead, enjoy some mashed cauliflower.

Foods to Avoid

The Limited "Bad" Fats

You need to be aware of unhealthy, processed trans fats, and polyunsaturated fats. These fats are acquired through processing and are found in foods, including fast foods, crackers, margarine, and cookies. Avoid canola, soybean, safflower, and cottonseed vegetable oils. If the oil was processed in a factory and prepackaged, you need to be aware of its fat content.

Processed Foods

Don't purchase any items if you see carrageenan on the label. Like so many other people, you shouldn't feel too guilty if you crave all of those processed foods. It happens!

Generally, look for labels with the least amount of ingredients. Usually, the ones that provide the most nutrition are listed in those shorter lists.

Here are just a few of the items you may not realize are loaded with carbs: Bread, pasta, pizza crusts, or crackers and cookies made with these grains:

- Barley: 44 carbs - 4 protein - 1 gram of fat
- Buckwheat: 33 carbs - 6 protein - 1 gram of fat

- Corn: 32 carbs - 4 protein - 1 gram of fat
- Millet: 41 carbs - 6 protein - 2 grams fat
- Oats: 36 carbs - 6 protein - 3 grams fat
- Rice: 45 carbs - 5 protein - 2 grams fat
- Rye: 15 carbs - 3 protein - 1 gram of fat

Watch out for the Sugar Products also:

- Raw Sugar: 12 grams of carbs
- High-Fructose Corn Syrup: 14 grams of carbs
- Honey: 17 grams of carbs
- Maple Syrup: 14 grams of carbs
- Cane Sugar: 12 grams of carbs
-

Some of the foods are surprising because they were deemed for years as a healthy and nutritious snack. I bet you see a few of the culprits that will beckon you onto the wrong path:

- Cereal Bars
- Rice Cakes
- Protein Bars
- Potato Chips
- Flavored Nuts
- Popcorn
- Pretzels
- Crackers

3.BENEFITS OF KETO DIET

Now, we get to the reason we are all here! What is it that the ketogenic diet can do for you? Luckily for you, there are a number of benefits this new lifestyle can bring to you. Whether you are looking to lose weight, balance your hormones, or just be healthier overall, the ketogenic diet may be your best option!

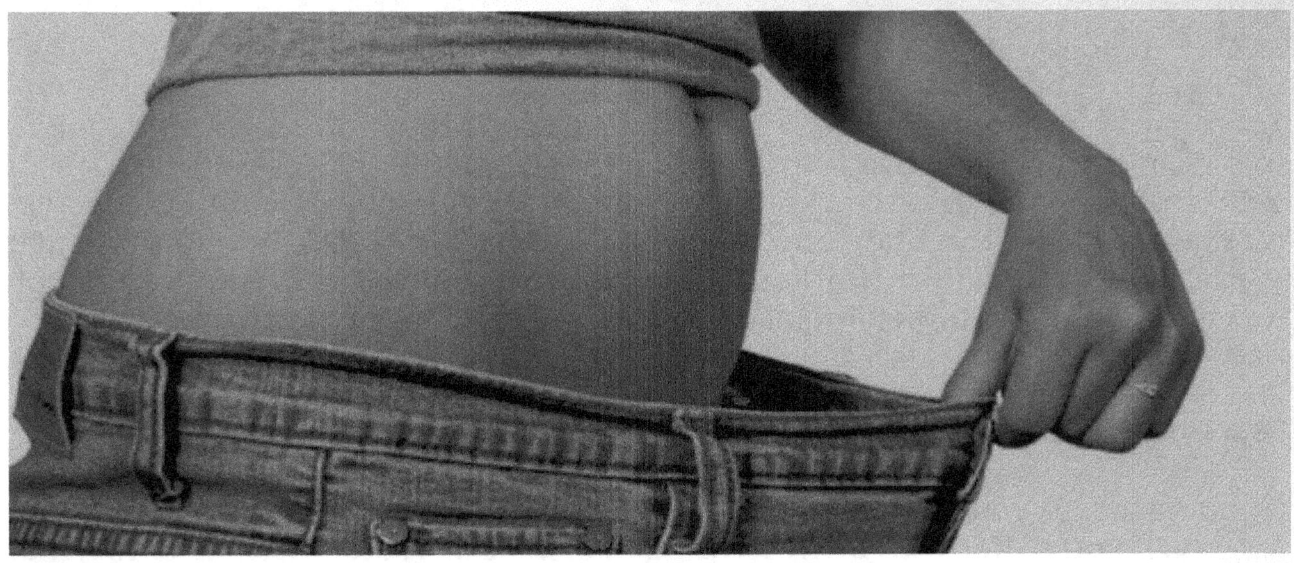

Weight Loss

Weight loss is one of the major reasons people begin the ketogenic diet in the first place. The idea of a high-fat, low-carb diet has been used for a very long time now. One of the major reasons the ketogenic diet works is due to the fact that this way of eating helps suppress appetite. As you lower your insulin levels by eating less carbs, you will be lowering the levels of fat in your body.
As you follow the ketogenic diet, you will be tapping into your own fat reserves as energy. Up until this point, your body has been using the easiest way to create energy from what it is given. From this point on, you will be retraining

your body to use fat as energy instead! It is a win-win situation for you as you begin to feel more energetic and burn fat at the same time. As you do this and combine with ketone supplements, you will be losing weight in no time.

Lower Blood Sugar for Type 2 Diabetes

As mentioned earlier, the ketogenic diet can help individuals lower their insulin levels. This is due to the fact that your body will be running off ketones instead of relying on glucose. As your body learns how to utilize fat and ketones for energy, this means that you will no longer need to worry about excess blood sugar levels or the need to get exogenous insulin.

Slows Down Aging

It almost sounds too good to be true, doesn't it? As you follow the ketogenic diet, it has been found that a low carb diet can lower the oxidative stress in the body. As this happens, it can increase one's lifespan. Studies show that as the insulin levels in the body lower, oxidative stress also lowers.

PCOS: Polycystic Ovary Syndrome

There are many women who suffer from PCOS. This syndrome is often linked to insulin resistance and in turn, causes a range of different hormonal issues for women. When following the ketogenic diet, this could help address the insulin resistance within the body and help those who have PCOS. In one particular study, they found that the ketogenic diet did help improve body weight, testosterone markets, fasting insulin, and the LH/FSH ratio for the women who had PCOS.

IBS: Irritable Bowel Syndrome

If you have IBS, you may think that a high-fat, low-carb diet could mean doom for you. If you suffer with symptoms such as bloating, stomach discomfort, or chronic diarrhea, the ketogenic diet may be able to actually help you in the long run! The long-term effects may be worth it if you are on the fence about the diet.
At first, upping fat can cause a bit of increased diarrhea, but as you lower your sugar consumption, this may help provide relief to symptoms caused by IBS. In fact, individuals have claimed that the ketogenic diet can improve stool habits, abdominal pain, and improves the overall quality of life thanks to a proper diet!

Increased Brain Function

While weight loss is a popular reason individuals begin the ketogenic diet, another major reason is improved brain function. Think about it; how often do you have a hard time focusing on simple tasks? Perhaps you go through your day, feeling exhausted, and leaning on high-carb foods to get you through. What if I told you that that high-sugar, high-carbohydrate foods were doing you more harm than good? Sure, they give you a burst of energy, but then they make you tired all over again AND make you fat. Through the ketogenic diet, you can improve your ability to learn, improve your memory recollection, and improve overall brain function.

According to Dr. Myhill, he found that through the ketogenic diet, the heart and the brain are able to run up to 25% more efficient when the body is running on ketones as opposed to blood sugar. In a study done on older adults following the ketogenic diet, they were able to improve their overall memory function, including their short term memory.

Increased Mitochondrial Function

Let's take a moment and go back to high school science. As you recall, the mitochondria are the energy factories in your cells. If the cells did not have the mitochondria, we would all be dead. This is why the health of your mitochondrial function is vital for your health, performance, immune function, and more. We are only as healthy as our mitochondria. Luckily on the ketogenic diet, you can increase the function of your mitochondria!

According to Dr. Gabriela Segura, she explains that the mitochondria functions better on the ketogenic diet due to the fact that the diet has the ability to increase energy levels in a more efficient way that is both stable and long-burning. Through diet, you gain the ability to increase energetic output while reducing the production of the free radicals that can be damaging to your system.

You see, the mitochondria were designed to specifically use fat for energy in the first place. As you use fat as the energy source, this helps decrease the toxic load and increase energy production. The key here is fat metabolism through ketone bodies by the liver. This process can only occur within your mitochondrion, which stimulates powerful anti-inflammatory antioxidants in your body. As you increase the overall health of your mitochondria, you will increase the health of your whole body!

Stabilize Energy Levels

Let me paint you a picture. You are sitting at your desk, and the clock strikes noon. At this point, your morning coffee begins to wear off, and you begin craving a little pick-me-up. That is your body craving energy and running out of glucose to run off of. As you begin to follow a ketogenic diet, you can say goodbye to your cravings for sugar and caffeine. While following a proper diet, you can keep your energy levels stable throughout the day and avoid the mid-afternoon slumps you may be experiencing at this point.

When your body is running on ketones, this is a readily available source of energy. As your body adapts to using this new source of energy, you will easily be able to get through your day without having energy level swings or food for that matter! Through consuming fewer calories, you can still lose weight and feel energetic at the same time!

Athletic Performance

The ketogenic diet is a very popular option for athletes due to enhanced endurance performance. While there have been many studies done on ketosis and sports performance, one, in particular, is known as the FASTER study. The results of this study showed that for those who followed a ketogenic diet, they had more mitochondria compared to the control group. This meant that these individuals had lower lactate load, lower oxidative stress, and were fueled off fat for a higher-intensity workout.

Epilepsy

Fun fact, the ketogenic diet has been used since the 1900s to treat patients who had epilepsy. In fact, this diet is still used widely as therapy for children who have seizures and uncontrolled epilepsy. While following this diet, patients typically are able to take fewer medications and still have better control over the symptoms.

Alzheimer's

As more research is being completed on the ketogenic diet, scientists are starting to believe that the ketogenic diet could have a major effect on those who have Alzheimer's. In fact, some scientists refer to this disease as Type 3 diabetes due to the fact that as this happens, the brain loses its ability to utilize glucose, leading to high levels of inflammation. While this poses as an issue, under the proper diet, the brain could still be able to function on ketones. It is still being studied closely, but it could be a step in the proper direction.

Cancer

Another growing belief in the science community is that ketosis could be a key prevention of cancer. This may be due to the fact that cancer cells survive on glucose as a fuel source. On the ketogenic diet, individuals deprive the cancer cells of the glucose in the first place and can starve out the cancer in the process. While it is still being studied, it is becoming more popular for individuals who are being treated for several different types of cancer.

While these are some of the major benefits of the ketogenic diet, the list can go on for a very long while and is becoming longer as researchers complete more studies of the diet to have a better understanding. The ketogenic diet can also benefit:

- Heartburn
- Fatty Liver Disease
- Migraines
- Mood Stabilization
- Parkinson's Disease
- Epilepsy
- And more!

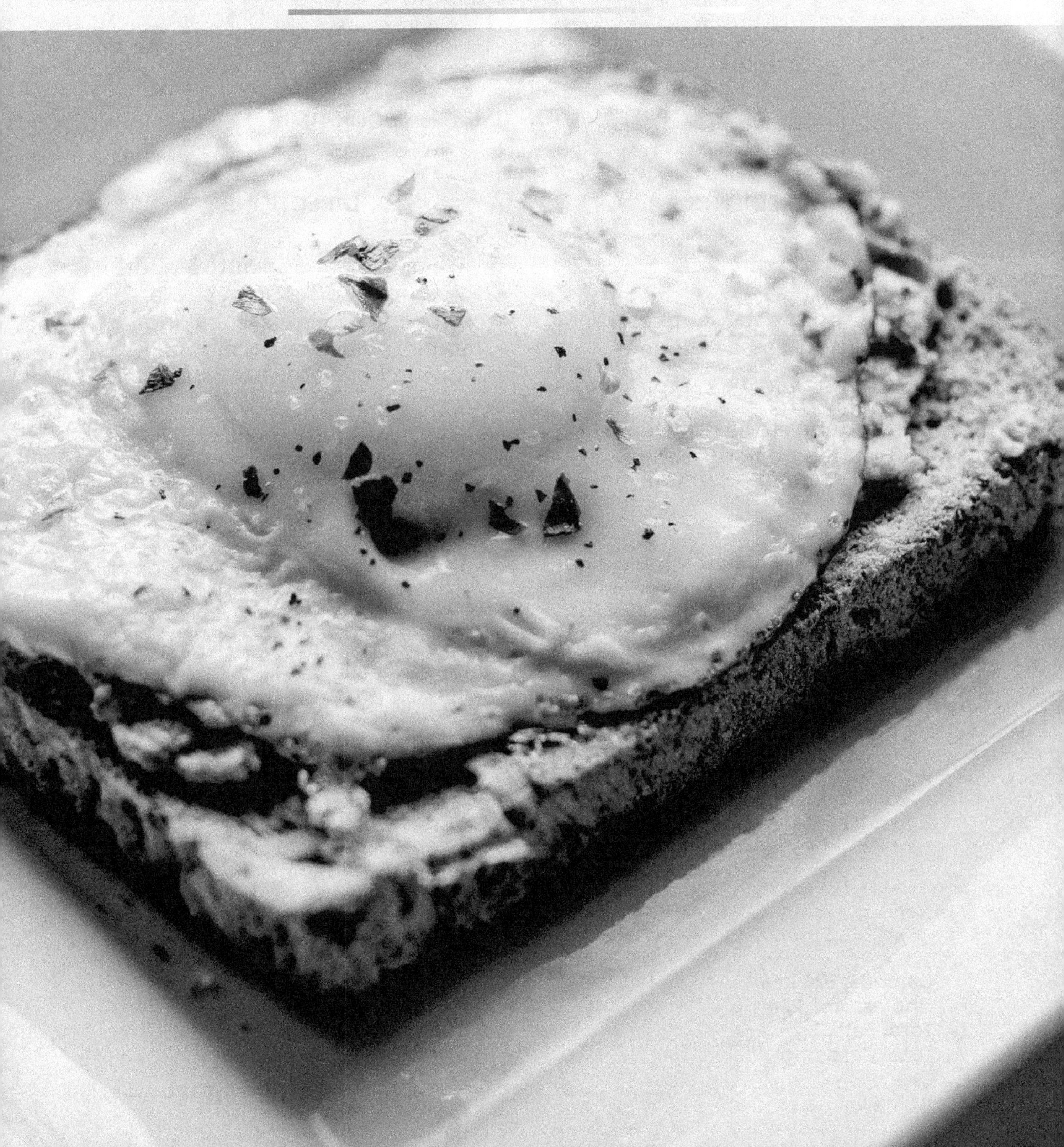

4. BREAKFAST

1. GREEN BANANA PANCAKES

PREPARATION TIME
20'

COOK TIME
15'

SERVING
4

INGREDIENTS

- 2 large peeled bananas
- 2 eggs
- 6 tablespoons coconut flour
- 2 teaspoons cassava flour or arrowroot starch
- Pinch salt
- ¼ teaspoon stevia powder
- 1 tablespoon baking powder
- Coconut oil grass-fed butter

DIRECTIONS

1. Puree the banana until smooth.
2. Mix the coconut flour, stevia, arrowroot or cassava, baking soda, and the pinch of salt in a mixing bowl to make a powder mixture.
3. Whisk egg lightly in a small bowl, then pour into the banana, mix well.
4. Then add the powder mixture to it. If the mixture is too thick, add some water with a spoon to make it slightly thin; do not over-water.
5. Preheat a skillet along with butter, ghee, or oil.
6. Pour in the batter in the skillet with a spoon.
7. When it is golden brown from the top, flip it, cook until brown, and take out on a plate. Serve hot.

NUTRITIONS

- Calories: 224 kcal
- Cholesterol: 224mg
- Total Fat: 32g
- Total Carbs: 5g

2. BERRY BREAD SPREAD

PREPARATION TIME
15'

COOK TIME
0

SERVING
3

INGREDIENTS

- 2 cups coconut cream
- 2 ounces strawberries
- 1 ½ ounce blueberries
- 1 ½ ounce raspberries
- ½ teaspoon coconut extract

DIRECTIONS

1. Dice three of each berry in small pieces separately.
2. Blend the remaining strawberries, blueberries, and raspberries in a blender until smooth.
3. Mix in the coconut extract and coconut cream.
4. Blend again until smooth, and then add in the diced berries.
5. Serve chilled.

NUTRITIONS

- Calories: 285 kcal
- Total Fat: 18g
- Total Carbs: 5.5g
- Protein: 6.8g

3. CHOCOLATE BREAD SPREAD

PREPARATION TIME
15'

COOK TIME
1'

SERVING
3

INGREDIENTS

- 4 cups sweet cream
- 2 ounces coconut oil
- 3 ounces chocolate
- 1 teaspoon coconut extract
- 1 tablespoon powdered cacao
- Groundnuts (optional)

DIRECTIONS

1. Put sweet cream in a microwavable bowl and heat for 10-15 seconds
2. Add in coconut oil and mix, then mix in the chocolate and powdered cacao. Mix well
3. Heat the mixture in the microwave for a few minutes
4. When it is warm, if you like, you can add groundnuts
5. Pour in fridge bowls, and chill
6. Serve as you desire

NUTRITIONS

- Calories: 257 kcal
- Total Fat: 19g
- Total Carbs: 7.5g
- Protein: 11.8g

4. KETO ALMOND CEREAL

PREPARATION TIME	**COOK TIME**	**SERVING**
20'	5'	3

INGREDIENTS

- 3 cups unsweetened coconut flakes
- 1 cup sliced almonds
- ¾ tablespoon cinnamon
- ¾ tablespoon nutmeg

DIRECTIONS

1. Preheat the oven to 250°F
2. Mix the almonds and coconut flakes together, and then add the nutmeg and cinnamon. Mix well
3. Spread the nut mixture on a baking tray, and bake for 3-5 minutes
4. Take out when slightly brown
5. Enjoy with milk

NUTRITIONS

- Calories: 104 kcal
- Fat: 15g
- Carbohydrates: 4g
- Protein: 5g

5. KETO GRANOLA CEREAL

PREPARATION TIME
30'

COOK TIME
5'

SERVING
3

INGREDIENTS

- 1 cup flaxseeds
- A Large egg
- 1 cup Almonds
- 1 cup Hazelnuts
- 1 cup Pecans
- 1/3 cup Pumpkin seeds
- 1/3 cup Sunflower seeds
- 1/4 cup melted butter or coconut oil or ghee for dairy-free
- 1 tsp. Vanilla extract

DIRECTIONS

1. Preheat the oven to 370°F, and line the baking drays with wax or parchment paper
2. Pulse the almonds and hazelnuts in a food processor intermittently until chopped into smaller and larger pieces, then add pecans and chop again into smaller and larger pieces. You will later add Pecans since they are softer
3. Add the pumpkin seeds, sunflower seeds, and flaxseeds, and pulse just until everything is mixed well. Don't over-process; you should have most seeds in intact form
4. Whisk an egg white and pour it into the food processor
5. Then, whisk together the melted butter and vanilla extracts in a small bowl, and evenly pours that in the food processor, too
6. Pulse again to mix well until it combines in the form of coarse meal and nut pieces, and everything should be a little moist from the egg white and butter.
7. Transfer the mixture to the prepared baking tray, evenly pressing, bake for 15 to 18 minutes, or until slightly brown from the edges.
8. Let it cool, and then break it into pieces.

NUTRITIONS

- Calories: 441 kcal
- Fat: 40g
- Carbohydrates: 4g
- Protein: 16g

6. KETO FRUIT CEREAL

PREPARATION TIME

20'

COOK TIME

5'

SERVING

3

INGREDIENTS

- 1 cup coconut flakes
- ½ cup sliced strawberries
- ¼ cup sliced raspberries

DIRECTIONS

1. Preheat oven to 300°F.
2. Prepare a baking tray with parchment paper
3. Slice the berries into small bits.
4. Spread the coconut flakes on the tray, bake for 5 minutes until brown from the edges.
5. Take out the baked coconut cereals, let it cool.
6. Then add in sliced raspberries and strawberries.
7. Enjoy with almond milk.

NUTRITIONS

- Calories: 201 kcal
- Fat: 44g
- Carbohydrates: 4g
- Protein: 19g

7. KETO CHICKEN AND AVOCADO

PREPARATION TIME
20'

COOK TIME
5'

SERVING
1

INGREDIENTS

- 6 medium-sized pieces of chicken Boneless.
- 1 avocado
- 2 eggs
- Keto Mayo
- Salt
- Pepper
- Ground Garlic
- ⅛ cup olive oil

DIRECTIONS

1. Soft boil 2 eggs, and slice them in half, so you have four pieces.
2. Put the seasonings together in a bowl and stir well.
3. Sprinkle them generously on the chicken pieces, cover, and let it sit for 5 minutes.
4. Heat the olive oil in a pan, and fry the chicken until cooked, remove from the flame and set aside.
5. Remove the pit from the avocado dice in half and set aside.
6. Sprinkle a little salt on the avocados (optional).
7. Spread mayo on the chicken (optional).
8. On a plate, set your eggs, chicken, and avocados. Enjoy hot.

NUTRITIONS

- Calories: 441 kcal
- Fat: 64g
- Carbohydrates: 9g
- Protein: 23g

8. KETO ALMOND PANCAKE

 **PREPARATION TIME**
30'

 **COOK TIME**
10'

 **SERVING**
1

INGREDIENTS

- 1 ½ cups almond flour
- 3 teaspoons baking powder
- 1 teaspoon salt
- 1 tablespoon stevia
- 1 ¼ cup almond milk
- 1 egg
- 3 tablespoons melted ghee
- 2 teaspoons olive oil

DIRECTIONS

1. Put in dry the ingredients and stir.
2. In another bowl, mix the egg, ghee, and milk together.
3. Mix the dry ingredients with the wet ingredients, whisk well, until no lumps.
4. Heat a frying pan and pour in olive oil to the pan one teaspoon at a time for each pancake.
5. Pour in the batter and brown each side equally.
6. Serve warm.

NUTRITIONS

- Calories: 430 kcal
- Fat: 19g
- Carbohydrates: 3g
- Protein: 21g

9. KETO MEATBALLS

PREPARATION TIME	COOK TIME	SERVING
30'	20'	3

INGREDIENTS

- 11 eggs
- 7 ounces mozzarella cheese
- 4 ounces chopped and cooked bacon
- 3 chopped scallions
- 1 ounce ground beef
- Salt
- Pepper
- A teaspoon olive oil

DIRECTIONS

1. Preheat the oven to 350°F and grease the muffin tray with oil.
2. Put the scallions evenly in the tin at the bottom.
3. In a bowl, mix the eggs and add a teaspoon of oil.
4. Add in the cheese, salt and pepper to taste. Mix well.
5. In another bowl, mix the bacon and the chicken together.
6. Add this meat mixture into cheese and stir well until combined.
7. Pour the mix into the muffin tray and bake for 17-20 minutes.
8. Serve hot.

NUTRITIONS

- Calories: 632 kcal
- Fat: 43g
- Carbohydrates: 15g
- Protein: 49g

10. KETO SCRAMBLED EGGS

PREPARATION TIME
10'

COOK TIME
5'

SERVING
41

INGREDIENTS

- 3 eggs
- 1 ounce ghee
- Salt and pepper

DIRECTIONS

1. Whisk the eggs, then add salt and pepper to taste. Mix well.
2. Heat the oil in a skillet and pour in the egg mixture and scramble until you cook the eggs.
3. Serve hot.

NUTRITIONS

- Calories: 148 kcal
- Fat: 15g
- Carbohydrates: 1.3g
- Protein: 12g

11. KETO FLAXSEED BREAD

PREPARATION TIME
1 HOUR

COOK TIME
35'

SERVING
6

INGREDIENTS

- 7 egg whites
- 2 egg yolks
- 6 tablespoons coconut oil or olive oil
- 3 cups flaxseed
- 3 sachets Stevia
- 3 teaspoons baking powder
- 1 teaspoon salt
- ½ cups water

DIRECTIONS

1. Preheat the oven to 350°F.
2. Pour in the egg whites, egg yolks, flaxseed, Stevia, oil, salt, water, and baking powder in a mixing bowl, and mix well with a wooden spoon.
3. Put into a blender and blend for 2-3 minutes. You can use a hand mixer too.
4. Grease a baking pan and line it with parchment paper.
5. Pour the batter into the pan, and bake for 30 minutes.
6. Take out from the oven and let it cool on a cake rack before slicing it.

NUTRITIONS

- Calories: 199 kcal
- Total Fat: 39g
- Total Carbs: 8g
- Protein: 15g

12. KETO OMELET

PREPARATION TIME
10'

COOK TIME
5'

SERVING
1

INGREDIENTS

- 3 large eggs
- Salt and pepper
- ½ ounce butter
- 4 sliced mushrooms
- ½ ounce olive oil
- 1 ounce shredded parmesan cheese
- 1 small chopped onion

DIRECTIONS

1. Whisk the eggs and season with salt and pepper, then mix well.
2. Heat the oil or butter in a frying pan.
3. Add in the mushrooms and onions and sauté until onions become soft.
4. Pour in the egg mixture.
5. When the egg mixture is firm, then sprinkle cheese on top.
6. When the bottom is cooked, flip with a spatula, cook from another side.
7. Take out the omelet on a serving plate and enjoy.

NUTRITIONS

- Calories: 550 kcal
- Fat: 37g
- Carbohydrates: 06.7g
- Protein: 24g

13. KETO BACON AND EGGS

PREPARATION TIME
10'

COOK TIME
5'

SERVING
1

INGREDIENTS

- 3 eggs
- Salt and pepper
- 3 spoons shredded cheese
- 5 ounces sliced bacon
- 3 spoons olive oil
- 3 spoons ghee
- Cherry tomatoes
- Fresh parsley

DIRECTIONS

1. Whisk the eggs and season with salt and pepper.
2. Heat the ghee and oil together in a pan. Put in the bacon and sauté for 1 to 2 minutes and take it out and set aside. Pour the eggs into the same pan to cook in the drippings.
3. Turn off the heat and toss in the cheese to melt.
4. Add the bacon and stir. Serve warm.

NUTRITIONS

- Calories: 212 kcal
- Fat: 20.3g
- Carbohydrates: 5g
- Protein: 19g

14. TACOS WITH BACON AND GUACAMOLE

PREPARATION TIME	**COOK TIME**	**SERVING**
15'	5'	2

INGREDIENTS

- 3 tablespoons diced cooked sweet potatoes
- 2 slices cooked uncured all-natural bacon
- 2 eggs
- 1 tablespoon Brain Octane Oil
- 1 tablespoon grass-fed ghee
- 1 medium organic avocado
- ¼ cup chopped romaine lettuce
- ¼ teaspoon Himalayan pink salt
- Micro cilantro

DIRECTIONS

1. Crack an egg without piercing the yolk then set it aside.
2. Heat a small skillet at medium heat level, and then add a tablespoon of ghee.
3. Pour in your egg and pierce the yolk, then cook from both sides for a minute or two. It should be solid, but not overcooked. Take out on a paper towel
4. Repeat the process with the second egg. You'll now have two yolks that will serve as the cages for your taco.
5. Mash the avocado in a bowl with light hands. When it's half done, add Brain Octane oil and Himalayan pink salt.
6. Spread the avocado mix evenly on each part of the eggs, then place chopped romaine lettuce evenly on both tacos.
7. Spread the diced sweet potatoes evenly on both sides, and put a strip of bacon on each side.
8. Place your micro cilantro evenly, then sprinkle some Himalayan pink salt, and fold in half. Enjoy!

NUTRITIONS

- Calories: 387 kcal
- Protein: 11g
- Carbs: 9g
- Fiber: 5g
- Fat: 35g

15. CHICKEN AVOCADO SALAD

PREPARATION TIME
40'

COOK TIME
40'

SERVING
4

INGREDIENTS

- 1 pound boneless chicken thighs
- 4 tablespoons extra virgin olive oil
- 3 tablespoons chopped celeries
- 2 tablespoons cilantro
- 1 large ripe avocado
- 1 ½ teaspoon oregano
- 1 tablespoon lemon juice
- ½ cup almond milk, ½ cup diced onion
- ½ teaspoon pepper

DIRECTIONS

1. Pour in the almond milk in a bowl, add in the oregano, and then stir well.
2. Slice up the boneless chicken thighs and rub the slices with the almond milk mixture. Let it sit for 13 to 15 minutes. Preheat the oven to 300°F, and line the baking tray with a foil sheet.
3. Place the coated chicken slices on the baking tray and bake for 30 to 40 minutes.
4. Meanwhile, slice the avocado into cubes, drizzle some olive oil and lemon juice, then set it aside.
5. In a salad bowl, mix in the cilantro, chopped celeries, and onion, and sprinkle some pepper. Take out the chicken and garnish it with the avocado mix and salad.
6. Serve warm.

NUTRITIONS

- Calories: 256 kcal
- Total Fat: 49g
- Total Carbs: 8g
- Protein: 19g

PREPARATION TIME
40'

COOK TIME
10'

SERVING
4

INGREDIENTS

- 4 ounces cream cheese cut into chunks
- 3 sliced red baby bell peppers
- 3 tablespoons onion salt
- 2 cups shredded mozzarella cheese low moisture
- 2 tablespoons grass-fed butter or other healthy fat
- 2 eggs
- 2 tablespoons no sugar added ketchup
- 2 tablespoons Keto mayo
- 1 sliced yellow onion
- 1 teaspoon garlic powder
- 1 teaspoon Italian seasoning
- 1 tablespoon onion salt
- 1 teaspoon sea salt
- 1 ½ cups almond flour
- 1 sliced jalapeno
- 1 teaspoon sea salt
- 1 teaspoon ground parsley
- 1 teaspoon black pepper
- I pound shaved steak
- 1 tablespoon Lime Juice
- 1 tablespoon Sriracha
- Mayo Sauce

DIRECTIONS

1. Whisk the eggs and set aside.
2. Pour the mozzarella and cream cheese into a microwave-safe bowl, and place it in a microwave for half a minute. Use a spoon or spatula to mix the mozzarella and cream cheese well.
3. Add the garlic powder, Italian seasoning, and the onion salt to the bowl, then the beaten egg and the almond flour, and mix thoroughly until firm like yellowish dough. Set aside the mixture.
4. Thinly slice your shaved meat. Melt the butter in a preheated skillet on medium heat.
5. Add the onions, peppers, and sauté until tender.
6. Add the shaved meat and sauté until brown.
7. Take off the skillet and immediately pour in the American cheese and cover. The heat will melt it. After 4 to 5 minutes, stir the contents of the skillet thoroughly.
8. Take out the dough and divide it into 10 to 12 balls, or depending on your desired size. Flatten each ball with the help of a rolling pin.
9. Disperse the meat mixture, ensuring enough space to seal.
10. Fold the flattened dough in half and use a fork to seal the edges.
11. Heat the frying oil. When hot enough, carefully place the pockets inside, and fry until golden brown from each side. In another bowl, mix the lime juice, No-Sugar-Added Ketchup, sriracha, and mayo. Use a fork to mix well. Spread in pockets before serving.

NUTRITIONS

- Carbs: 7.5g
- Calories: 439 kcal
- Total Fat: 52.2g
- Protein: 12.7g

17. LOW CARB CAESAR SALAD

PREPARATION TIME	COOK TIME	SERVING
20'	0	4

INGREDIENTS

- 1 head romaine lettuce
- 6 slices cooked and diced bacon
- ½ cup shredded parmesan cheese
- 5 tablespoons grated parmesan cheese
- 3 teaspoons Worcestershire sauce
- 2 teaspoons fresh lemon juice
- 2 minced anchovy fillets, or anchovy sauce
- 2/3 cup Keto mayonnaise
- ¼ cup sour cream
- 1 minced garlic clove
- 1 teaspoon mustard powder
- Black pepper

DIRECTIONS

1. Slice the lettuce, and mix with the cheese and bacon like a normal salad.
2. For the dressing, put all the ingredients in a single bowl and mix well.
3. Set down your salad and top with as much dressing as you want. Enjoy!

NUTRITIONS

- Calories: 112 kcal
- Total Fat: 32g
- Total Carbs: 5.0g
- Protein: 14.3g

18. KETO CAULIFLOWER AND EGGS

PREPARATION TIME
20'

COOK TIME
5'

SERVING
4

INGREDIENTS

- 5 hard-boiled eggs
- 2 stalks celery
- 1 ½ cups Greek yogurt
- ¼ teaspoon pepper
- 1 head cauliflower
- 1 tablespoon white vinegar
- 1 tablespoon yellow mustard
- 1 teaspoon salt
- 1 cup water
- ¾ white onion, diced

DIRECTIONS

1. Chop the cauliflower into bite-size pieces, and place it in a pot with a cup of water.
2. Drain the cauliflower and set aside
3. Dice up the boiled eggs, mix them into the cauliflower.
4. Dice the celery and onion, and then add in the cauliflower and egg mixture.
5. Add the Greek yogurt, pepper, white vinegar, yellow mustard salt, and the diced white onion to the mixture, and mix well with a wooden spoon.
6. Dish with salt and serve.

NUTRITIONS

- Calories: 224 kcal
- Total Fat: 22g
- Total Carbs: 8.2g
- Protein: 23.5 g

19. ZUCCHINI PIZZA BITES T

 **PREPARATION TIME** 30'

 **COOK TIME** 10'

 **SERVING** 4

INGREDIENTS

- 4 large zucchinis
- 1 cup tomato sauce
- 2 teaspoon oregano
- 4 cups mozzarella cheese
- ½ cup parmesan cheese
- Low carb pizza toppings of your choice

DIRECTIONS

1. Slice your zucchinis into small pieces, in a quarter of an inch or less.
2. Preheat the oven to 450°F.
3. Line a baking pan or tray with foil, set it aside.
4. Place zucchini pieces in the pan. Top them with tomato sauce, cheese, oregano, and other low carb toppings you like. Bake for five minutes, and then broil for five minutes more. Serve warm.

NUTRITIONS

- Calories: 231 kcal
- Protein: 26.7g
- Carbs: 4.8g
- Fat:: 74g

20. EGG ON AVOCADO

PREPARATION TIME
20'

COOK TIME
5'

SERVING
3

INGREDIENTS

- 1 ½ teaspoon garlic powder
- ¾ teaspoons sea salt
- 1/3 cup Parmesan cheese
- ¼ teaspoon black pepper
- 4 avocados
- 6 small eggs

DIRECTIONS

1. Preheat muffin tins to 350°F.
2. Slice the avocado into half, and take the seed out. Mix the pepper, salt, and garlic well.
3. Generously season your avocado with the above seasoning mix.
4. Place the seasoned avocado in the muffin tin; side with the empty hollow facing up.
5. Whisk the egg and gently pour in each avocado. If you doubt that the avocado has enough space, lightly scrape the inside.
6. Finally, sprinkle cheese on top of the avocado. Repeat the process for all, and then bake for 15 minutes and Serve hot.

NUTRITIONS

- Calories: 364 kcal
- Total Carbs: 2.5g
- Total Fat: 55.5g
- Protein: 13.5g

21. BACON & EGG BREAKFAST MUFFINS

PREPARATION TIME
15'

COOK TIME
30'

SERVING
12

INGREDIENTS

- 8 large eggs
- 8 slices bacon
- 6 cup green onion

DIRECTIONS

1. Warm the oven to 350°F. Spray the muffin tin wells using a cooking oil spray. Chop the onions and set aside.
2. Prepare a large skillet using the medium temperature setting. Fry the bacon until it's crispy and place on a layer of paper towels to drain the grease. Chop it into small pieces after it has cooled.
3. Whisk the eggs, bacon, and green onions, mixing well until all of the fixings are incorporated. Add the egg mixture into the muffin tin (halfway full). Bake it for about 20 to 25 minutes. Cool slightly and serve.

NUTRITIONS

- Calories: 69 kcal
- Carbohydrates: 0.4g
- Protein: 5.6g
- Fats: 4.9g

5. LUNCH RECIPES

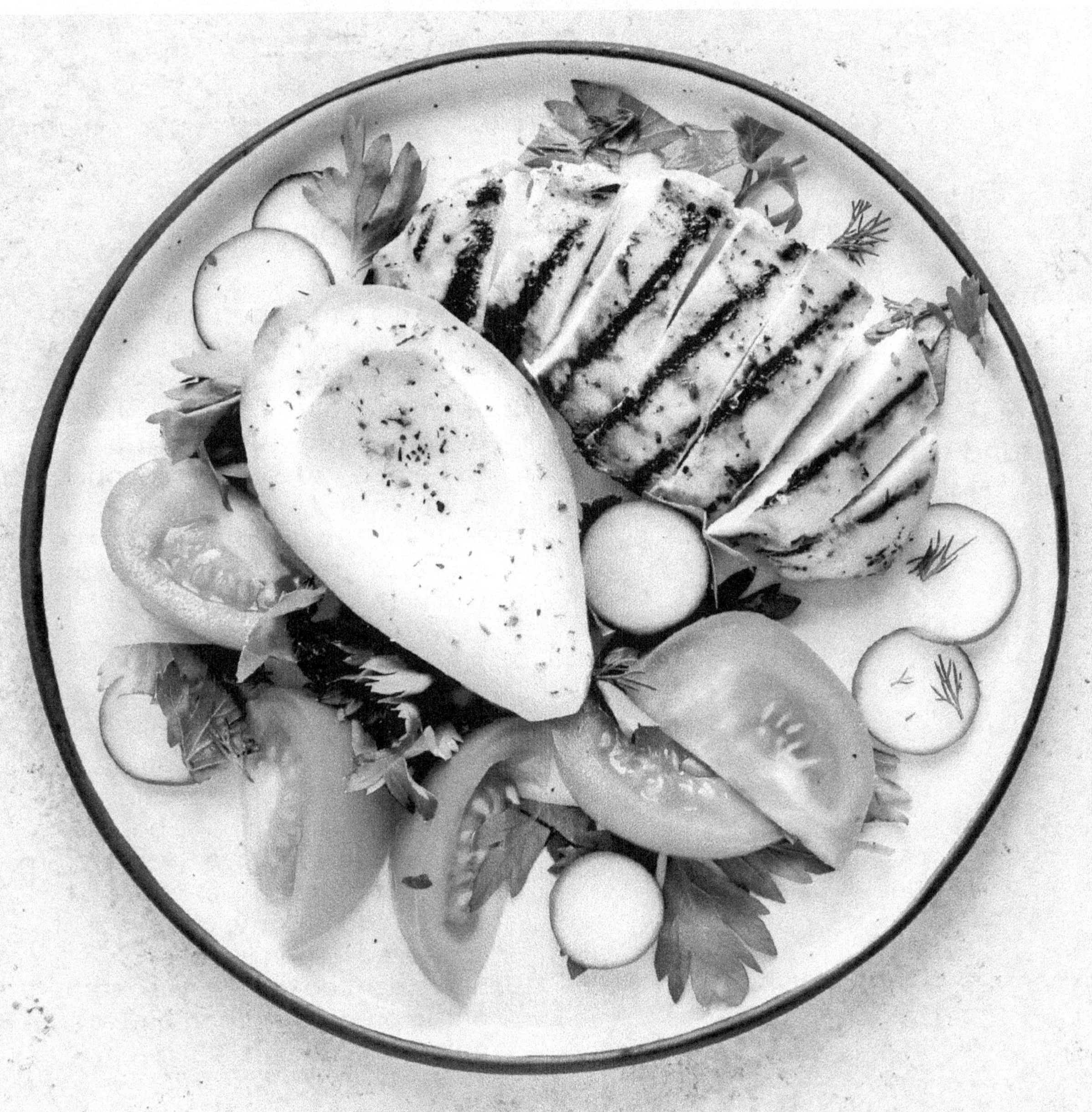

1. KETO BAKED SALMON WITH LEMON AND BUTTER

PREPARATION TIME
10'

COOK TIME
30'

SERVING
3

INGREDIENTS

- 1 pound salmon
- 1 lemon
- 3 oz. butter
- 1 tablespoon olive oil
- Ground black pepper and sea salt to taste

DIRECTIONS

1. Grease a large-sized baking dish with the olive oil and preheat your oven to 400°F.
2. Place the salmon in the baking dish, preferably skin-side down. Generously season with pepper and salt to taste.
3. Thinly slice the lemon and place the slices over the salmon. Cover the fish with ½ of the butter, preferably in very thin slices.
4. Bake until the salmon flakes easily with a fork and is opaque (for 25 to 30 minutes) on the middle rack.
5. Now, over moderate heat in a small sauce pan; heat the remaining butter until it begins to bubble. Immediately remove the pan from heat; set aside and let cool a bit. Gently add in some of the freshly squeezed lemon juice.
6. Serve the cooked fish with some of the prepared lemon butter and enjoy.

NUTRITIONS

- Calories: 576 kcal
- Total Fat: 46g
- Saturated Fat: 22g
- Total Carbohydrates: 1.3g
- Dietary Fiber: 0.4g
- Sugars: 0.4g
- Protein: 31g

2. CURRY ROASTED CAULIFLOWER

PREPARATION TIME
5'

COOK TIME
15'

SERVING
2

INGREDIENTS

- 1/2 pound cauliflower, approximately a large head; remove the outer leaves, cut into half and then cut out and discard the core; cutting it further into bite-sized pieces
- 2 tablespoons nuts; any of your favorites
- 1 ½ teaspoon curry powder
- 1 tablespoon plus 1 teaspoon extra-virgin olive oil
- 2 teaspoons lemon juice, fresh
- 1 teaspoon kosher salt

DIRECTIONS

1. Preheat your oven to 425°F.
2. Toss the cauliflower pieces with olive oil in a large bowl until evenly coated. Sprinkle with curry powder and salt; give everything a good toss until nicely coated. Spread them out on a large-sized rimmed baking sheet, preferably in an even layer and transfer them to the preheated oven.
3. Roast for 8 to 10 minutes, until the bottom is starting to turn brown. Turn them over and continue to roast for 5 to 7 more minutes, until fork-tender. Place them in the bowl again; toss with the freshly squeezed lemon juice and your favorite nuts. Serve immediately and enjoy.

NUTRITIONS

- Calories: 188 kcal
- Total Fat: 16.7g
- Saturated Fat: 1.8g
- Total Carbohydrates: 8.1g
- Dietary Fiber: 6g
- Sugars: 4.8g
- Protein: 6.3g

3. LEMON ROSEMARY CHICKEN THIGHS

PREPARATION TIME
10'

COOK TIME
45'

SERVING
4

INGREDIENTS

- 4 chicken thighs
- 2 garlic cloves, roughly chopped
- 4 sprigs Rosemary, fresh
- 1 lemon, medium
- 2 tablespoons butter
- Pepper, and salt to taste

DIRECTIONS

1. Preheat your oven to 400F° in advance and heat up a cast-iron skillet over high heat as well.
2. Season both sides of the meat with pepper, and salt. When the skillet is hot; carefully place the coated thighs, preferably skin side down into the hot skillet, and sear them for 4 to 5 minutes, until nicely brown.
3. Carefully flip and flavor the thighs with the lemon juice (only use ½ of the lemon). Quarter the leftover lemon halves and throw the pieces into the pan with the chicken.
4. Add the chopped garlic cloves together with some rosemary into the skillet.
5. Place the skillet inside the oven and bake for 30 minutes.
6. Remove the skillet from the oven. To add flavor, moisture, and more crispiness; add a portion of butter over the chicken thighs. Bake for 10 more minutes.
7. Serve hot and enjoy.

NUTRITIONS

- Calories: 159 kcal
- Total Fat: 8.8g
- Saturated Fat: 4.3g
- Total Carbohydrates: 6.9g
- Dietary Fiber: 3g
- Sugars: 3.2g
- Protein: 13.9g

4. KETO GROUND BEEF AND GREEN BEANS

PREPARATION TIME	COOK TIME	SERVING
5'	10'	2

INGREDIENTS

- 1 ½ ounces butter
- 8 ounces green beans, fresh, rinsed and trimmed
- 10 ounces ground beef
- 1/4 cup crème fraîche or home-made mayonnaise, optional
- Pepper and salt to taste

DIRECTIONS

1. Over moderate heat in a large, frying pan; heat a generous dollop of butter until completely melted.
2. Increase the heat to high and immediately brown the ground beef until almost done (5 minutes.) Sprinkle with pepper and salt to taste.
3. Decrease the heat to medium; add more butter and continue to fry the beans in the same pan with the meat for 5 more minutes, stirring frequently.
4. Season the beans with pepper and salt as well. Serve with the leftover butter and add in the optional crème fraîche or mayonnaise, if desired.

NUTRITIONS

- Calories: 513 kcal
- Total Fat: 44g
- Saturated Fat: 23.5g
- Total Carbohydrates: 8.5g
- Dietary Fiber: 3.6g
- Sugars: 4g
- Protein: 30g

5. ROASTED BRUSSELS SPROUTS WITH PECANS AND ALMOND BUTTER

PREPARATION TIME
5'

COOK TIME
35ì

SERVING
4

INGREDIENTS

- 1 pound Brussels sprouts, fresh; ends trimmed
- ¼ cup almond butter
- 2 tablespoons olive oil
- ½ cup pecans, chopped or to taste
- Fresh ground black pepper and salt to taste

DIRECTIONS

1. Using a pastry brush; lightly coat a large-sized roasting pan with 1 tablespoon olive oil and preheat your oven to 350°F in advance.
2. Cut each Brussels sprout lengthwise into halves or fourths.
3. Chop the pecans using a sharp knife and measure the desired amount out.
4. Put the chopped pecans and Brussels sprouts into a large-sized plastic bowl and toss with 1 tablespoon olive oil; generously season with fresh ground black pepper and salt to taste.
5. Arrange the pecans and Brussels sprouts in a single layer on a roasting pan. Roast in the preheated oven until the sprouts begin to brown on the edges and are fork-tender, for 30 to 35 minutes, stirring several times during the cooking process.
6. Just before serving, toss the cooked pecans and Brussels sprouts with almond butter. Serve hot and enjoy.

NUTRITIONS

- Calories: 175 kcal
- Total Fat: 23.5g
- Saturated Fat: 3.1
- Total Carbohydrates: 11g
- Dietary Fiber: 5.7g
- Sugars: 2.9g
- Protein: 7.6g
-

6. SPICY BEEF MEATBALLS

PREPARATION TIME
10'

COOK TIME
10'

SERVING
3

INGREDIENTS

- 1 cup mozzarella or cheddar cheese; cut into 1x1 cm cubes
- 1 pound minced ground beef
- 1 teaspoon olive oil
- 3 tablespoons parmesan cheese
- 1 teaspoon garlic powder
- ½ teaspoon each pepper, and salt

DIRECTIONS

1. Thoroughly combine the ground beef with the entire dry ingredients; mix well.
2. Wrap the cheese cubes into the mince; forming 9 meatballs from the prepared mixture.
3. Pan-fry the formed meatballs until cooked through, covered (uncover and stirring frequently).

NUTRITIONS

- Calories: 595 kcal
- Total Fat: 44g
- Saturated Fat: 20.5g
- Total Carbohydrates: 2.8g
- Dietary Fiber: 0.1g
- Sugars: 0.2g
- Proteins: 49g

7. KETOGENIC SPICY OYSTER

 **PREPARATION TIME** 10'

 **COOK TIME** 5'

 **SERVING** 2

INGREDIENTS

- 12 oysters shucked
- 1 tablespoon olive oil
- 7-8 basil leaves, fresh
- 1 tablespoon garlic chili paste
- ⅛ teaspoon salt

DIRECTIONS

1. Combine the olive oil with the garlic chili paste and salt in a medium-size mixing bowl; mix well.
2. Add the oysters into the prepared sauce; turning them several times until thoroughly coated.
3. Create a bed for the oysters to cook by spreading the basil leaves out on an oven-safe dish.
4. Transfer the oysters and sauce over the bed of basil leaves; spreading them in a single layer on the dish.
5. Turn on the broiler over high heat.
6. Place the dish on the top rack (approximately a few inches away from the broiler) and broil for a few minutes.
7. Once done; immediately remove them from the oven. Serve hot and enjoy.

NUTRITIONS

- Calories: 102 kcal
- Total Fat: 8g
- Saturated Fat: 2.5g
- Total Carbohydrates: 2g

- Dietary Fiber: 0g
- Sugars: 0.3g
- Protein: 4g

8. GARLIC LIME MAHI-MAHI

PREPARATION TIME
15'

COOK TIME
10' + 30' MARINATION

SERVING
4

INGREDIENTS

- 4 Mahi-Mahi filets (approximately 1 to 1 ¼ pounds)
- Zest and juice 1 large lime, fresh
- ¼ cup avocado oil
- 3 cloves garlic, minced
- ⅛ teaspoon each ground black pepper and fine grain sea salt

DIRECTIONS

For Marinade:

1. Thoroughly combine the entire ingredients (except the filets) together in a small-sized mixing bowl. Pour the mixture on top of filets in a large zip-lock bag or large shallow dish. Let marinate for 30 minutes, at room temperature.
2. Pour the marinade into a large sauté pan (preferably with a cover) and heat it over medium heat at 390°F. Once hot; carefully add the filets into the hot pan; cover and cook the filets for a couple of minutes, until cooked through.
3. Immediately remove the sauté pan from heat; set aside and let rest for 5 minutes, covered. Serve warm and enjoy.

NUTRITIONS

- Calories: 248 kcal
- Total Fat: 14g
- Saturated Fat: 1.7g
- Total Carbohydrates:0.7g
- Dietary Fiber: 0.1g
- Sugars: 0g
- Protein: 24g

9. FISH AND LEEK SAUTÉ

PREPARATION TIME
15'

COOK TIME
10'

SERVING
2

INGREDIENTS

- 1 leek, chopped
- 2 trout fillets, diced (approximately 8 oz.)
- 1 tablespoon tamari soy sauce
- 1 teaspoon ginger, grated
- 1 tablespoon avocado oil
- Salt to taste

DIRECTIONS

1. Over moderate heat in a large skillet; heat the avocado oil until hot. Once done; add and sauté the chopped leek for a few minutes, until turn soften.
2. Immediately add the diced trout with grated ginger, tamari sauce, and salt to taste.
3. Continue to sauté the trout until it's not translucent anymore and cooked through.
4. Serve immediately and enjoy.

NUTRITIONS

- Calories: 175 kcal
- Total Fat: 7.6g
- Saturated Fat: 1.5g
- Total Carbohydrates: 5.2g
- Dietary Fiber: 0.8g
- Sugars: 1.7g
- Protein: 21g

10. KETO BAKED SALMON WITH PESTO

PREPARATION TIME
10'

COOK TIME
30'

SERVING
2

INGREDIENTS

- 1 ounce. green pesto
- ½ pound salmon
- Pepper and salt, to taste

For Green sauce:
- ¼ cup Greek yogurt
- 1ounce green pesto
- ¼ teaspoon garlic
- Pepper and salt, to taste

DIRECTIONS

1. Preheat your oven to 400°F.
2. Arrange the salmon in a well-greased baking dish, preferably skin-side down. Spread the pesto over the salmon and then, sprinkle with pepper and salt to taste.
3. Bake in the preheated oven until the salmon flakes easily with a fork (25 to 30 minutes.)
4. In the meantime, stir the entire sauce ingredients together in a large bowl. Serve the cooked fish with some of the prepared sauce and enjoy.

NUTRITIONS

- Calories: 274 kcal
- Total Fat: 21g
- Saturated Fat: 3.9g
- Total Carbohydrates: 2.9g
- Dietary Fiber: 0.6g
- Sugars: 1.7g
- Protein: 26g

11. ROASTED SALMON WITH PARMESAN DILL CRUST

 **PREPARATION TIME**
10'

 **COOK TIME**
10'

 **SERVING**
2

INGREDIENTS

- ½ pound salmon; cut into pieces
- 1 tablespoon dill weed
- ¼ cup cottage cheese
- 1 tablespoon olive oil
- ¼ cup parmesan cheese, grated

DIRECTIONS

1. Preheat the oven to 450°F.
2. Combine cottage cheese with parmesan cheese, olive oil, and dill in a large-sized mixing bowl; mix well.
3. Line a large-sized baking sheet with aluminum foil and then, arrange the salmon pieces on it.
4. Smear ½ of the cottage cheese mixture over the salmon.
5. Roast in the preheated oven until the fish flakes easily and the crust is brown, for 10 minutes.
6. Serve the cooked fish with the remaining prepared sauce and enjoy.

NUTRITIONS

- Calories: 352 kcal
- Total Fat: 22g
- Saturated Fat: 6.6g
- Total Carbohydrates: 5.7g
- Dietary Fiber: 1.5g
- Sugars: 0.5g
- Protein: 33g

12. KETO FRIED SALMON WITH BROCCOLI AND CHEESE

PREPARATION TIME
15'

COOK TIME
25'

SERVING
3

INGREDIENTS

- ¾ pound salmon; cut into pieces
- 3 tablespoons butter
- ½ pound broccoli; cut into small florets
- 2 ounces cheddar cheese, grated
- Pepper and salt, to taste
- 1 lime

DIRECTIONS

1. Preheat your oven using the broiler settings, to 400°F.
2. Let the broccoli florets to simmer for a couple of minutes, preferably in lightly salted water. Ensure that the broccoli maintains its delicate color and chewy texture; drain well.
3. Now arrange the broccoli in a baking dish, preferably well-greased. Add the butter and pepper to taste.
4. Sprinkle with cheese and bake in the preheated oven until the cheese turns golden in color, for 15 to 20 minutes.
5. Now, over moderate heat in a large saucepan; heat the butter until completely melted and fry the salmon pieces for a couple of minutes per side. Serve the pan-fried salmon with baked broccoli and enjoy.

NUTRITIONS

- Calories: 392 kcal
- Total Fat: 25g
- Saturated Fat: 11.8g
- Total Carbohydrates: 5.8g
- Dietary Fiber: 3.4g
- Sugars: 1.4g
- Protein: 31g

13. KETO RIB EYE STEAK

PREPARATION TIME
5'

COOK TIME
20'

SERVING
2

INGREDIENTS

- ½ pound grass-fed rib-eye steak, preferably 1" thick
- 1 teaspoon Adobo Seasoning
- 1 tablespoon extra-virgin olive oil
- Pepper and sea salt, to taste

DIRECTIONS

1. Add steak in a large-sized mixing bowl and drizzle both sides with a small amount of olive oil. Dust the seasonings on both sides; rubbing the seasonings into the meat.
2. Let sit for a couple of minutes and heat up your grill in advance. Once hot; place the steaks over the grill, and cook until both sides are cooked through (15 to 20 minutes) flipping occasionally.

NUTRITIONS

- Calories:257 kcal
- Total Fat: 19g
- Saturated Fat: 5g
- Total Carbohydrates: 0.3g
- Dietary Fiber: 0.2g
- Sugars: 0g
- Protein: 24g

14. EGGLESS SALAD

PREPARATION TIME
5'

COOK TIME
5'

SERVING
4

INGREDIENTS

- 1 stalk celery, chopped
- Vegan mayonnaise, as required
- 1 pound extra firm tofu
- 2 tablespoons onions, minced
- Pepper and salt, to taste

DIRECTIONS

1. Mash the tofu into a chunky texture, just like an egg salad.
2. Add the mayonnaise until you get your desired consistency.
3. Add in the leftover ingredients; stir well.
4. Serve on keto pitas or keto bread, with vegetables and enjoy.

NUTRITIONS

- Calories: 117 kcal
- Total Fat: 7.8g
- Saturated Fat: 1.3g
- Total Carbohydrates: 2.8g
- Dietary Fiber: 1.5g
- Sugars: 1.4g
- Protein: 16g

15. MOUTH-WATERING GUACAMOLE

PREPARATION TIME	COOK TIME	SERVING
5'	0	6

INGREDIENTS

- 3 avocados, pitted
- ¼ cup cilantro, freshly chopped, plus more for garnish
- Juice of 2 limes
- ½ teaspoon kosher salt
- 1 small jalapeño, minced
- ½ small white onion, finely chopped

DIRECTIONS

1. Combine the avocados with cilantro, lime juice, jalapeño, onion, and salt in a large-sized mixing bowl; mix well.
2. Give the ingredients a good stir and then, slowly turn the bowl; running a fork through the avocados. Once you get your desired level of consistency, immediately season it with more salt, if required. Just before serving; feel free to garnish your recipe with more fresh cilantro.

NUTRITIONS

- Calories: 165 kcal
- Total Fat: 15g
- Saturated Fat:: 2.1g
- Total Carbohydrates: 9.5g
- Dietary Fiber: 6.9g
- Sugars: 1.1g
- Protein: 2.1g

16. SMOKED SALMON SALAD

PREPARATION TIME
5'

COOK TIME
0

SERVING
1

INGREDIENTS

- 2 ounces smoked salmon
- 1 lemon slice
- 4 olives
- 1 teaspoon pink peppercorns, crushed lightly
- 1 handful arugula salad leaves, fresh

DIRECTIONS

1. Place the olives and salad leaves into a large plate or shallow bowl.
2. Arrange the smoked salmon over the salad.
3. Sprinkle the top of smoked salmon with lightly crushed pink peppercorns.
4. Garnish your salad with a lemon slice; serve immediately and enjoy.

NUTRITIONS

- Calories: 149
- Total Fat: 5.2g
- Saturated Fat: 1.4g
- Total Carbohydrates: 4g
- Dietary Fiber: 1.7g
- Sugars: 3.4g
- Protein: 11g

17. ZUCCHINI CAULIFLOWER FRITTERS

 **PREPARATION TIME** 5'

 **COOK TIME** 15'

 **SERVING** 2

INGREDIENTS

- ¼ head cauliflower, chopped (roughly 1 ½ cups)
- 1 tablespoon coconut oil
- ⅛ cup coconut flour
- 1 medium zucchini; grated
- Black pepper and sea salt, to taste

DIRECTIONS

1. Steam the cauliflower until just fork tender (3 to 5 minutes). Add cauliflower to your food processor and process on high power until broken down into very small chunks (ensure it's not mashed.)
2. Squeeze the moisture as much as possible from the grated veggies using a nut milk bag or dishtowel.
3. Transfer to a large bowl along with the grated zucchini and add flour coconut flour followed by pepper, salt, and any seasonings you desire; combine well. Make 4 small-sized patties from the mixture.
4. Now, over moderate heat in a large pan; heat 1 tablespoon of coconut oil. Work in batches and cook the fritters for 2 to 3 minutes per side. The cooked fritters can be served with some dipping sauce of your choice on side.

NUTRITIONS

- Calories: 112 kcal
- Total Fat: 8g
- Saturated Fat: 5.8g
- Total Carbohydrates: 5.6g
- Dietary Fiber: 2.2
- Sugars: 2g
- Protein: 2.1g

18. ROASTED GREEN BEANS

PREPARATION TIME
5'

COOK TIME
30'

SERVING
4

INGREDIENTS

- 3 cups green beans, raw, trimmed
- 1 tablespoon Italian seasoning
- 2 tablespoons olive oil
- Ground black pepper and kosher salt to taste
- 4 tablespoons pumpkin seeds

DIRECTIONS

1. Combine the green beans with olive oil and seasonings in a large bowl; toss to coat. Spread them out on a roasting pan or cookie sheet, preferably large-sized.
2. Roast in the oven for 20 minutes at 400°F.
3. Remove; give everything a good stir.
4. Place the cookie sheet again into the oven and roast for 10 more minutes. Remove; sprinkle the pumpkin seeds, serve warm and enjoy.

NUTRITIONS

- Calories: 155 kcal
- Total Fat: 12g
- Saturated Fat: 2.7g
- Total Carbohydrates: 8.7g
- Dietary Fiber: 3.7g
- Sugars: 3.5g
- Protein: 6.4g

19. BACON BLEU ZOODLE SALAD

PREPARATION TIME	**COOK TIME**	**SERVING**
5'	0'	2

INGREDIENTS

- 4 cups zucchini noodles
- ½ cup bacon, cooked and crumbled
- 1 cup fresh spinach, chopped
- 1/3 cup bleu cheese, crumbled
- Fresh cracked pepper, to taste

DIRECTIONS

1. Toss the entire ingredients together in a large-sized mixing bowl.
2. Serve immediately, and enjoy.

NUTRITIONS

- Calories: 214 kcal
- Total Fat: 17g
- Saturated Fat: 2.9g
- Total Carbohydrates: 6g
- Dietary Fiber: 3.1g
- Sugars: 4.7g
- Protein: 33g

20. GARLIC BAKED BUTTER CHICKEN

PREPARATION TIME
10'

COOK TIME
40'

SERVING
4

INGREDIENTS

- 1 tablespoon rosemary leaves, fresh
- 3 chicken breasts, boneless, skinless (approximately 12 ounces); washed and cleaned
- 1 stick butter (½ cup)
- ½ cup Italian cheese, low fat and shredded
- 6 garlic cloves, minced
- Fresh ground pepper and salt to taste

DIRECTIONS

1. Grease a large-sized baking dish lightly with a pat of butter, and preheat your oven to 375°F.
2. Season the chicken breasts with pepper and salt to taste; arrange them in the prepared baking dish, preferably in a single layer; set aside.
3. Now, over medium heat in a large skillet; heat the butter until melted, and then cook the garlic until lightly browned, for 4 to 5 minutes, stirring every now and then. Keep an eye on the garlic; don't burn it.
4. Add the rosemary; give everything a good stir; remove the skillet from heat.
5. Transfer the already prepared garlic butter over the meat.
6. Bake in the preheated oven for 30 minutes.
7. Sprinkle cheese on top and cook until the cheese is completely melted, for a couple of more minutes.
8. Remove from the oven and let it stand for a couple of minutes. Transfer the cooked meat to large serving plates. Serve and enjoy.

NUTRITIONS

- Calories: 375 kcal
- Total Fat: 27g
- Saturated Fat: 16g
- Total Carbohydrates: 2.3g
- Dietary Fiber: 0.5g
- Sugars: 0.1g
- Protein: 30g

21. TURKEY AND RADISHES DLE SALAD

PREPARATION TIME
5'

COOK TIME
12'

SERVING
4

INGREDIENTS

- 1 tablespoon olive oil
- 1 pound radishes, trimmed and quartered
- 1 pound cooked turkey, chopped
- 1 onion, small, chopped
- ½ cup beef broth
- Pepper and salt to taste

DIRECTIONS

1. Over medium-high heat settings in a large saucepan; heat a tablespoon of olive oil.
2. Once hot; add and sauté the onion for a couple of minutes and then add the radishes; continue to sauté for 5 more minutes.
3. Add in the beef broth; give everything a good stir until evenly mixed. Cover the pan loosely and cook until the liquid is reduced and the radishes are fork-tender, for 5 minutes.
4. Add in the cooked turkey; season with pepper and salt to taste; giving everything a good stir. Serve immediately and enjoy.

NUTRITIONS

- Calories: 304 kcal
- Total Fat: 16g
- Saturated Fat: 4.3g
- Total Carbohydrates: 6.5g
- Dietary Fiber: 2.1g
- Sugars: 2.9g
- Protein: 31g
-

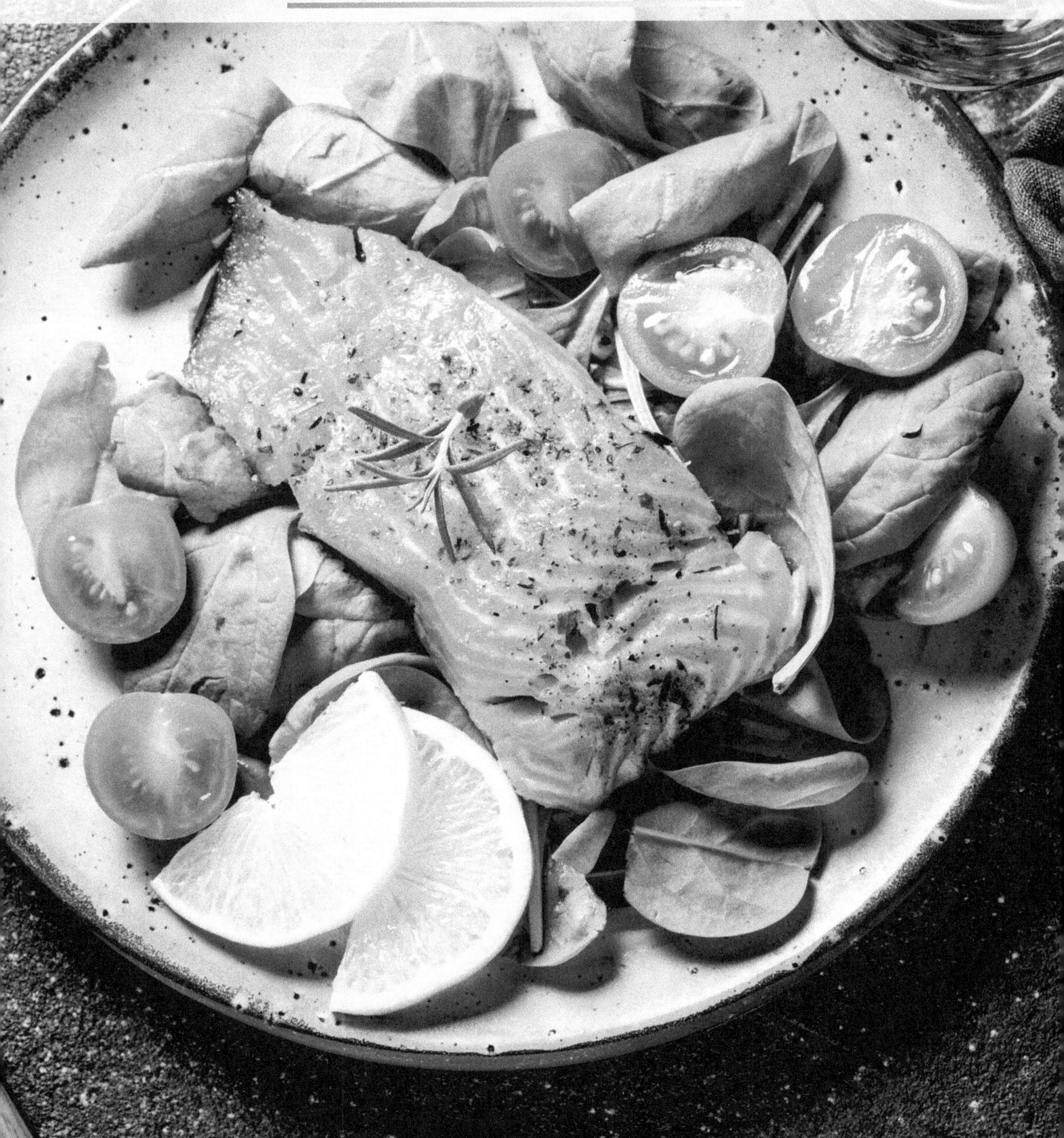

6. DINNER RECIPES

1. GRILLED PESTO SALMON WITH ASPARAGUS

 **PREPARATION TIME**
5'

 **COOK TIME**
15'

 **SERVING**
4

INGREDIENTS

- 4 (6-ounce) boneless salmon fillets
- Salt and pepper
- 1 bunch asparagus, ends trimmed
- 2 tablespoons olive oil
- ¼ cup basil pesto

DIRECTIONS

1. Preheat the grill to heat, and oil the grills.
2. Season the salmon with salt and pepper and sprinkle with spray to cook.
3. Grill the salmon on each side for 4 to 5 minutes, until cooked.
4. Throw the asparagus with oil and grill for about 10 minutes, until tender.
5. Spoon the salmon with the pesto, and serve with the asparagus.

NUTRITIONS

- Calories: 300 kcal
- Fat: 17.5g
- Protein: 34.5g
- Carbohydrates: 2.5g

2. SPICY SHRIMP AND SAUSAGE SOUP

PREPARATION TIME
15'

COOK TIME
30'

SERVING
4

INGREDIENTS

- 1 tablespoon olive oil
- 3 small stalks celery, diced
- 1 small yellow onion, chopped
- 1 small red pepper, chopped
- 3 cloves garlic, minced
- 1 tablespoon tomato paste
- 2 teaspoons smoked paprika
- ½ teaspoon ground coriander
- Salt and pepper
- 8 ounces chorizo sausage, diced
- 1 cup diced tomatoes
- 4 cups chicken broth
- 12 ounces shrimp, peeled and deveined
- Fresh chopped cilantro

DIRECTIONS

1. Heat up the oil over medium to high heat in a large stockpot.
2. Add the celery, onion, and red pepper, then sauté until tender for 6 to 8 minutes.
3. Then add the garlic, tomato paste, and seasonings and cook for 1 minute.
4. Add the tomatoes and sausage, and cook for 5 minutes.
5. Stir in the broth, then cook, uncovered, for 20 minutes and bring to a simmer.
6. Set seasoning to taste and then add the shrimp.
7. Simmer for about 3 to 4 minutes, until just cooked through.
8. In cups, spoon in and serve with fresh cilantro.

NUTRITIONS

- Calories: 465 kcal
- Fat: 28.5g
- 39 g of protein
- Fiber: 2g
- Net Carbs: 9.5g
-

3. CHEDDAR-STUFFED BURGERS WITH ZUCCHINI

PREPARATION TIME
10'

COOK TIME
15'

SERVING
4

INGREDIENTS

- 1 pound ground beef (80% lean)
- 2 large eggs
- ¼ cup almond flour
- 1 cup shredded cheddar cheese
- Salt and pepper
- 2 tablespoons olive oil
- 1 large zucchini, halved and sliced

DIRECTIONS

1. In a cup, add the beef, egg, almond flour, cheese, salt, and pepper.
2. Mix well, then shape into 4 even-sized patties.
3. Heat up the oil over medium to high heat in a large skillet.
4. Add the burger patties, and cook until browned for 5 minutes.
5. Flip the patties onto the skillet and add the zucchini, tossing to cover with grease.
6. Add salt and pepper and boil for 5 minutes, stirring the mixture.

NUTRITIONS

- Calories: 350 kcal
- Fat: 25g
- Protein: 43.5g
- Carbs: 10g
- Fiber: 4g
- Net Carbs: 9g

PREPARATION TIME
10'

COOK TIME
45'

SERVING
4

INGREDIENTS

- 4 boneless chicken breast halves (about 12 ounces)
- 4 slices deli ham
- 4 slices Swiss cheese
- 1 large egg, whisked well
- 2 ounces pork rinds
- ¼ cup almond flour
- ¼ cup grated parmesan cheese
- ½ teaspoon garlic powder
- Salt and pepper
- 2 cups cauliflower florets

DIRECTIONS

1. Preheat the oven to 350 ° F and add a foil on a baking sheet.
2. Sandwich the breast half of the chicken between parchment parts and pound flat.
3. Spread the bits out and cover with ham and cheese sliced over.
4. Roll the chicken over the fillings and then dip into the beaten egg.
5. In a food processor, mix the pork rinds, almond flour, parmesan, garlic powder, salt and pepper, and pulse into fine crumbs.
6. Roll the rolls of chicken in the mixture of pork rind then put them on the baking sheet.
7. Throw the cauliflower into the baking sheet with the melted butter and fold.
8. Bake for 45 minutes until the chicken is fully cooked.

NUTRITIONS

- Calories: 420 kcal
- Fat 23.5g
- Protein: 45g
- Carbohydrates: 7g
- Fiber: 2.5

5. SESAME-CRUSTED TUNA WITH GREEN BEANS

PREPARATION TIME
15'

COOK TIME
5'

SERVING
4

INGREDIENTS

- ¼ cup white sesame seeds
- ¼ cup black sesame seeds
- 4 (6 ounces) ahi tuna steaks
- Salt and pepper
- 1 tablespoon olive oil
- 1 tablespoon coconut oil
- 2 cups green beans

DIRECTIONS

1. In a shallow dish, mix the two kinds of sesame seeds.
2. Season the tuna with pepper and salt.
3. Dredge the tuna in a mixture of sesame seeds.
4. Heat up to high heat the olive oil in a skillet, then add the tuna.
5. Cook for 1 to 2 minutes until it turns seared, then sear on the other side.
6. Remove the tuna from the skillet, and let the tuna rest while using the coconut oil to heat the skillet.
7. Fry the green beans in the oil for 5 minutes then use sliced tuna to eat.

NUTRITIONS

- Calories: 380 kcal
- Fat: 19g
- Protein: 44.5g
- Carbs: 8g
- Fiber: 3g
- Net Carbs: 5g

6. CHOPPED KALE SALAD WITH BACON DRESSING

PREPARATION TIME
15'

COOK TIME
/

SERVING
2

INGREDIENTS

- 6 slices uncooked bacon
- 2 tablespoons apple cider vinegar
- 1 teaspoon Dijon mustard
- Liquid stevia, to taste
- Salt and pepper
- 4 cups fresh chopped kale
- ¼ cup thinly sliced red onion

DIRECTIONS

1. Cook the bacon in a skillet until the crisp is removed and sliced in paper towels.
2. In the skillet save ¼ cup of bacon grease and cover at low heat.
3. Whisk vinegar, mustard, and stevia in the apple cider then season with salt and pepper.
4. Throw in the kale and cook for 1 minute and then break between two plates.
5. Finish the salads and serve with red onion and chopped bacon.

NUTRITIONS

- Calories: 230 kcal
- Fat: 12g
- Protein: 15 g
- Carbs: 16g
- Fiber: 2.5g
- Net Carbs: 13.5g

7. KALE CAESAR SALAD WITH CHICKEN

PREPARATION TIME
10'

COOK TIME
10'

SERVING
2

INGREDIENTS

- 1 tablespoon olive oil
- 6 ounces boneless chicken thigh, chopped
- Salt and pepper
- 3 tablespoons mayonnaise
- 1 tablespoon lemon juice
- 1 anchovy, chopped
- 1 teaspoon Dijon mustard
- 1 clove garlic, minced
- 4 cups fresh chopped kale

DIRECTIONS

1. Heat up the oil over medium to high heat in a skillet.
2. Season with salt and pepper to the chicken then add to the skillet.
3. Cook until the chicken is not pink anymore, then remove from heat.
4. In a blender, add the mayonnaise, lemon juice, anchovies, mustard, and garlic.
5. Smooth mix, and then sprinkle with salt and pepper.
6. Throw the kale with the dressing, then break into half and top with the chicken

NUTRITIONS

- Calories: 245 kcal
- Fat: 28 g
- Protein: 48.5 g
- Carbs: 4 g
- Fiber: 8 g
- Net Carbs: 2 g

8. ROSEMARY ROASTED PORK WITH CAULIFLOWER

PREPARATION TIME
10'

COOK TIME
20'

SERVING
4

INGREDIENTS

- 1 ½ pounds boneless pork tenderloin
- 1 tablespoon coconut oil
- 1 tablespoon fresh chopped rosemary
- Salt and pepper
- 1 tablespoon olive oil
- 2 cups cauliflower florets

DIRECTIONS

1. Rub the coconut oil into the pork, then season with the rosemary, salt, and pepper.
2. Heat up the olive oil over medium to high heat in a large skillet.
3. Add the pork on each side and cook until browned for 2 to 3 minutes.
4. Sprinkle the cauliflower over the pork in the skillet.
5. Reduce heat to low, then cover the skillet and cook until the pork is cooked through (8 to 10 minutes).
6. Slice the pork with cauliflower and eat.

NUTRITIONS

- Calories: 300 kcal
- Fat: 15.5 g
- Protein: 37 g
- Carbohydrates: 3g
- Fiber: 1.5g
- Net Carbs: 1.5g

9. CHICKEN TIKKA WITH CAULIFLOWER RICE

PREPARATION TIME
10'

COOK TIME
6 HOURS

SERVING
6

INGREDIENTS

- 2 pounds boneless chicken thighs, chopped
- 1 cup canned coconut milk
- 1 cup heavy cream
- 3 tablespoons tomato paste
- 2 tablespoons Garam masala
- 1 tablespoon fresh grated ginger
- 1 tablespoon minced garlic
- 1 tablespoon smoked paprika
- 2 teaspoons onion powder
- 1 teaspoon guar gum
- 1 tablespoon butter
- 1 ½ cup rice cauliflower

DIRECTIONS

1. Place the chicken in a slow cooker and then stir in the remaining ingredients, except for the butter and cauliflower.
2. Cover and cook for 6 hours on low heat until the chicken is cooked and the sauce is thickened.
3. Melt the butter over medium to high heat into a saucepan.
4. Remove the riced cauliflower, and cook until tender (6 to 8 minutes).
5. Serve cauliflower rice with chicken Tikka.

NUTRITIONS

- Calories: 485 kcal
- Fat: 32g
- Protein: 43g
- Fiber: 1.5g
- Net carbs: 5g

10. GRILLED SALMON AND ZUCCHINI WITH MANGO SAUCE

PREPARATION TIME
5'

COOK TIME
10

SERVING
4

INGREDIENTS

- 4 (6 ounces) boneless salmon fillets
- 1 tablespoon olive oil
- Salt and pepper
- 1 large zucchini, sliced into coins
- 2 tablespoons fresh lemon juice
- ½ cup chopped mango
- ¼ cup fresh chopped cilantro
- 1 teaspoon lemon zest
- ½ cup canned coconut milk

DIRECTIONS

1. Preheat a grill pan, and sprinkle it with cooking spray liberally.
2. Brush with olive oil to the salmon and season with salt and pepper.
3. Apply lemon juice to the zucchini, and season with salt and pepper.
4. Put the zucchini and salmon fillets on the grill pan.
5. Cook for 5 minutes then turn all over and cook for another 5 minutes.
6. Combine the remaining ingredients in a blender and combine to create a sauce.
7. Serve the side-drizzled salmon filets with mango sauce and zucchini.

NUTRITIONS

- Calories: 350 kcal
- Fat: 21.5g
- Protein: 35g
- Carbohydrates: 8g
- Sugar: 2g
- Net Carbs: 6g

11. SLOW-COOKER POT ROAST WITH GREEN BEANS

 **PREPARATION TIME**
10'

 **COOK TIME**
8 HOURS

 **SERVING**
8

INGREDIENTS

- 2 medium stalks celery, sliced
- 1 medium yellow onion, chopped
- 1 (3 pounds) boneless beef chuck roast
- Salt and pepper
- ¼ cup beef broth
- 2 tablespoons Worcestershire sauce
- 4 cups green beans, trimmed
- 2 tablespoons cold butter, chopped

DIRECTIONS

1. In a slow-cooking dish, add the celery and onion.
2. Put the frying pan on top and season with salt and pepper.
3. Whisk the beef broth and the Worcestershire sauce together then pour in.
4. Cover and cook for 8 hours on low heat, until the beef is very tender.
5. Bring the beef off on a cutting board and cut it into chunks.
6. Return the beef to the slow cooker and add the chopped butter and the beans.
7. Cover and cook for 20 to 30 minutes on warm, until the beans are tender.

NUTRITIONS

- Calories: 375 kcal
- Fat: 13.5g
- Protein: 53g
- Carbohydrates: 6g
- Fiber: 2 g
- Net Carbs: 4 g

12. BEEF AND BROCCOLI STIR-FRY

PREPARATION TIME
20'

COOK TIME
15'

SERVING
4

INGREDIENTS

- ¼ cup soy sauce
- 1 tablespoon sesame oil
- 1 teaspoon garlic chili paste
- 1 pound beef sirloin
- 2 tablespoons almond flour
- 2 tablespoons coconut oil
- 2 cups chopped broccoli florets
- 1 tablespoon grated ginger
- 3 cloves garlic, minced

DIRECTIONS

1. In a small bowl, whisk the soy sauce, sesame oil, and chili paste together.
2. In a plastic freezer bag, slice the beef and mix it with the almond flour.
3. Pour in the sauce and toss to coat for 20 minutes, then let it rest.
4. Heat up the oil over medium to high heat in a large skillet.
5. In the pan, add the beef and sauce and cook until the beef is browned.
6. Move the beef to the skillet sides, and then add the broccoli, ginger, and garlic.
7. Sauté until tender-crisp broccoli, then throw it all together and serve hot.

NUTRITIONS

- Calories: 350 kcal
- Fat: 19g
- Protein: 37.5 g
- Fiber: 2g

13. PARMESAN-CRUSTED HALIBUT WITH ASPARAGUS

PREPARATION TIME
10'

COOK TIME
15'

SERVING
4

INGREDIENTS

- 2 tablespoons olive oil
- ¼ cup butter, softened
- Salt and pepper
- ¼ cup grated Parmesan
- 1 pound asparagus, trimmed
- 2 tablespoons almond flour
- 4 (6 ounces) boneless halibut fillets
- 1 teaspoon garlic powder

DIRECTIONS

1. Preheat the oven to 400°F and line a foil-based baking sheet.
2. Throw the asparagus in olive oil and scatter over the baking sheet.
3. In a blender, add the butter, Parmesan cheese, almond flour, garlic powder, salt and pepper, and mix until smooth.
4. Place the fillets with the asparagus on the baking sheet, and spoon the Parmesan over the eggs.
5. Bake for 10 to 12 minutes, and then broil until browned (2 to 3 minutes).

NUTRITIONS

- Calories: 415 kcal
- Fat: 26g
- Protein: 42g
- Carbohydrates: 6g
- Fiber: 3g
- Net Carbs: 3g

14. HEARTY BEEF AND BACON CASSEROLE

PREPARATION TIME
25'

COOK TIME
30'

SERVING
8

INGREDIENTS

- 8 slices uncooked bacon
- 1 medium head cauliflower, chopped
- ¼ cup canned coconut milk
- Salt and pepper
- 2 pounds ground beef (80% lean)
- 8 ounces mushrooms, sliced
- 1 large yellow onion, chopped
- 2 cloves garlic, minced

DIRECTIONS

1. Preheat the oven to 37°F.
2. Cook the bacon in a skillet until it crisp, then drain and chop on paper towels.
3. Bring to boil a pot of salted water, and then add the cauliflower.
4. Boil until tender for 6 to 8 minutes then drain and add the coconut milk to a food processor.
5. Mix until smooth, then sprinkle with salt and pepper.
6. Cook the beef until browned in a pan, and then cut the fat away.
7. Remove the mushrooms, onion, and garlic, and then move to a baking platter.
8. Place on top of the cauliflower mixture and bake for 30 minutes.
9. Broil for 5 minutes on high heat, then sprinkle with bacon to serve.

NUTRITIONS

- Calories: 410 kcal
- Fat: 25.5g
- Protein: 37g
- Fiber: 3g

15. SESAME WINGS WITH CAULIFLOWER

PREPARATION TIME
5'

COOK TIME
30'

SERVING
4

INGREDIENTS

- 2 ½ tablespoons soy sauce
- 2 tablespoons sesame oil
- 1 ½ teaspoons balsamic vinegar
- 1 teaspoon minced garlic
- 1 teaspoon grated ginger
- Salt
- 1 pound chicken wing, the wings itself
- 2 cups cauliflower florets

DIRECTIONS

1. In a freezer bag, mix the soy sauce, sesame oil, balsamic vinegar, garlic, ginger, and salt, then add the chicken wings.
2. Coat flip, and then chill for 2 to 3 hours.
3. Preheat the oven to 400°F and line a foil-based baking sheet.
4. Spread the wings along with the cauliflower onto the baking sheet.
5. Bake for 35 minutes, and then sprinkle on to serve with sesame seeds.

NUTRITIONS

- Calories: 400 kcal
- Fat: 28.5g
- Protein: 31.5g
- Carbohydrates: 4g
- Fiber: 1.5g
- Carbs: 2.5g

16. FRIED COCONUT SHRIMP WITH ASPARAGUS

PREPARATION TIME
15'

COOK TIME
10'

SERVING
6

INGREDIENTS

- 1 ½ cups shredded unsweetened coconut
- 2 large eggs
- Salt and pepper
- 1 ½ pounds large shrimp, peeled and deveined
- ½ cup canned coconut milk
- 1 pound asparagus, cut into 2-inch pieces

DIRECTIONS

1. Pour the coconut onto a shallow platter.
2. Beat the eggs in a bowl with a little salt and pepper.
3. Dip the shrimp into the egg first, and then dredge with coconut.
4. Heat up coconut oil over medium-high heat in a large skillet.
5. Add the shrimp and fry over each side for 1 to 2 minutes until browned.
6. Remove the paper towels from the shrimp and heat the skillet again.
7. Remove the asparagus and sauté to tender-crisp with salt and pepper, and then serve with the shrimp.

NUTRITIONS

- Calories: 535 kcal
- Fat 38.5 g
- Protein: 29.5g
- Carbs: 18g
- Fiber: 10g
- Net Carbs: 8g

17. COCONUT CHICKEN CURRY WITH CAULIFLOWER RICE

PREPARATION TIME
15'

COOK TIME
30'

SERVING
6

INGREDIENTS

- 1 tablespoon olive oil
- 1 medium yellow onion, chopped
- 1 ½ pounds boneless chicken thighs, chopped
- Salt and pepper
- 1 (14-ounce) can coconut milk
- 1 tablespoon curry powder
- 1 ¼ teaspoon ground turmeric
- 3 cups riced cauliflower

DIRECTIONS

1. Heat the oil over medium heat, in a large skillet.
2. Add the onions, and cook for about 5 minutes, until translucent.
3. Stir in the chicken and season with salt and pepper-cook for 6 to 8 minutes, stirring frequently until all sides are browned.
4. Pour the coconut milk into the pan, then whisk in the curry and turmeric powder.
5. Simmer until hot and bubbling (15 to 20 minutes).
6. Meanwhile, steam the cauliflower rice until tender with a few tablespoons of water.
7. Serve the cauliflower rice over the curry.

NUTRITIONS

- Calories: 430 kcal
- Fat: 29g
- Protein: 33.5g
- Carbohydrates: 9g

13. SPICY CHICKEN ENCHILADA CASSEROLE

PREPARATION TIME
15'

COOK TIME
1 HOUR

SERVING
6

INGREDIENTS

- 2 pounds boneless chicken thighs, chopped
- Salt and pepper
- 3 cups tomato salsa
- 1 ½ cups shredded cheddar cheese
- ¾ cup sour cream
- 1 cup diced avocado

DIRECTIONS

1. Preheat the oven to 375°F and grate a saucepan.
2. Add salt and pepper to the chicken and pour into the oven.
3. Layer the chicken over the salsa and sprinkle with cheese.
4. Cover with foil then bake until the chicken is cooked for 60 minutes.
5. Serve with chopped avocado and sour cream.

NUTRITIONS

- Calories: 550 kcal
- Fat: 31.5g
- Protein: 54 g
- Carbohydrates: 12 g
- Fiber: 4 g
- Net Carbs: 8 g

19. WHITE CHEDDAR BROCCOLI CHICKEN CASSEROLE

PREPARATION TIME
15'

COOK TIME
30'

SERVING
6

INGREDIENTS

- 2 tablespoons olive oil
- 1 pound boneless chicken thighs, chopped
- 1 medium yellow onion, chopped
- 1 clove garlic, minced
- 1 ½ cups chicken broth
- 8 ounces cream cheese, softened
- ¼ cup sour cream
- 2 ½ cups broccoli florets
- ¾ cup shredded white cheddar cheese

DIRECTIONS

1. Preheat the oven to 350°F and grease a saucepan.
2. Heat up the oil over medium to high heat in a large skillet.
3. Add the chicken to brown and cook on each side for 2 to 3 minutes.
4. Stir in the garlic and onion, then season with salt and pepper.
5. Stir for four to five minutes until the chicken is cooked clean.
6. Pour into the broth of chicken, and then add the cream cheese and sour cream.
7. Simmer until melted the cream cheese, and then stir in broccoli.
8. Drop the mixture into the saucepan and sprinkle with cheese.
9. Bake until hot and bubbling (25 to 30 minutes).

NUTRITIONS

- Calories: 435 kcal
- Fat: 32g
- Protein: 29.5g
- Carbohydrates: 6g
- Fiber: 1.5g

20. SAUSAGE STUFFED BELL PEPPERS

PREPARATION TIME	COOK TIME	SERVING
15'	45'	4

INGREDIENTS

- 1 medium head cauliflower, chopped
- 1 tablespoon olive oil
- 12 ounces ground Italian sausage
- 1 small yellow onion, chopped
- 1 teaspoon dried oregano
- Salt and pepper
- 4 medium bell peppers

DIRECTIONS

1. Preheat the oven to 350° afterward.
2. Pulse the cauliflower into rice-like grains in a food processor.
3. Heat the oil in a skillet over medium heat and then add the cauliflower-cook until tender (6 to 8 minutes).
4. In a cup, spoon the cauliflower rice, then reheat the skillet.
5. Stir in the sausage, cook until browned, and then remove the fat.
6. Stir the cauliflower sausage, and then add the onion, oregano, salt, and pepper.
7. Slice the peppers from the tips, remove the seeds and pith, then spoon the sausage mixture.
8. Place the peppers in a baking dish upright, and then cover the platter with foil.
9. Bake for 30 minutes, then uncover and bake for another 15 minutes. Serve warm.

NUTRITIONS

- Calories: 355 kcal
- Fat: 23.5g
- Protein: 19g
- Carbohydrates: 16.5g
- Fiber: 6g
- Net Carbs: 10.5g

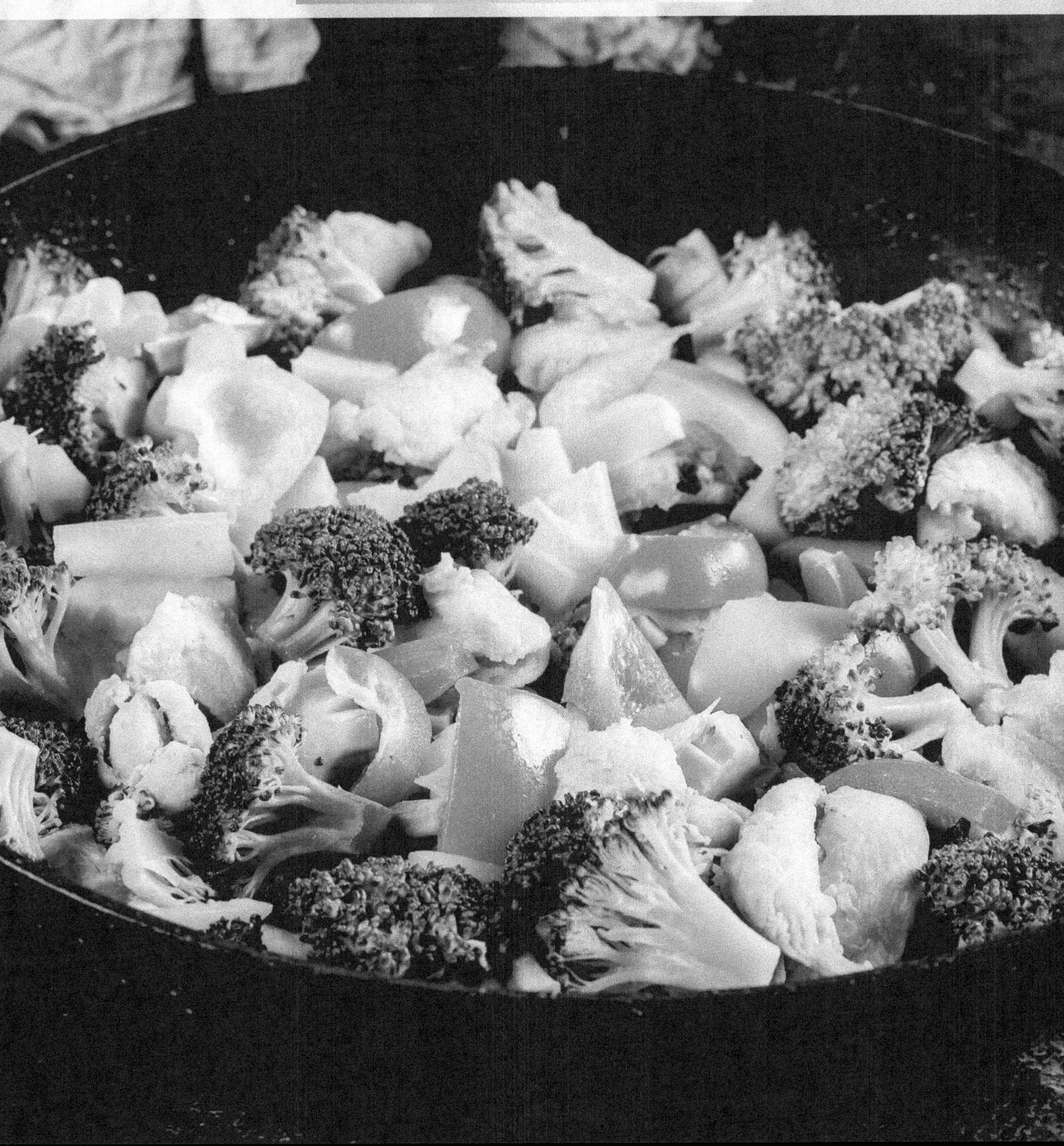

7. VEGETABLE RECIPES

1. KETO SPINACH ROLL

PREPARATION TIME
10'

COOK TIME
5

SERVING
15

INGREDIENTS

- 3 whole-wheat tortillas
- 10-ounces spinach, frozen
- ½ cup sour cream
- ½ cup mayonnaise

DIRECTIONS

1. In a medium, pan cooks your spinach over medium heat and drain.
2. Combine the sour cream, mayonnaise, and spinach in a mixing bowl.
3. Spread the creamy mixture evenly over tortillas, roll them up and keep them in the fridge overnight.
4. The next day cut into slices, serve and enjoy!

NUTRITIONS

- Calories: 73 kcal
- Cholesterol: 5mg
- Sugar: 0.6g
- Carbohydrates: 7.3g
- Protein: 1.7g
- Fat: 4.5g

2. ARTICHOKE AVOCADO SPINACH SALAD

PREPARATION TIME
15'

COOK TIME
0

SERVING
4

INGREDIENTS

- 4 cups spinach, fresh, washed
- 4 tablespoons lemon juice, fresh
- 1 avocado, peeled, diced
- ½ teaspoon garlic, minced
- ½ cup scallions, chopped
- 14 ounces artichoke hearts, drained, halved
- ¼ teaspoon pepper
- 1 teaspoon sugar or sugar substitute

DIRECTIONS

1. In a mixing bowl add the artichokes, spinach, scallions, and the avocado, toss well.
2. In a small bowl mix together garlic, sugar, lemon juice and pepper.
3. Pour the mix over the salad and serve fresh. Enjoy!

NUTRITIONS

- Calories: 168 kcal
- Fat: 10.2g
- Cholesterol: 0mg
- Sugar: 3g
- Carbohydrates: 18g
- Protein: 5.4g

3. CORN LIME AVOCADO SALAD

PREPARATION TIME
15'

COOK TIME
0

SERVING
6

INGREDIENTS

- 3 ears corn, cooked, cut kernels from cob
- 1 ripe avocado, peel, diced
- 1 garlic clove, minced
- 1 red bell pepper, cored, diced
- 1 jalapeno pepper, minced
- 1 scallion, sliced
- Pepper to taste
- 1 tablespoon lime juice, fresh
- 2 tablespoons olive oil

DIRECTIONS

1. In a mixing bowl add the scallion, garlic, corn, avocado, jalapeno, bell pepper and toss well.
2. In a small bowl, combine the lime juice with oil.
3. Pour the oil and juice mixture over salad and toss well. Season with pepper and serve fresh. Enjoy!

NUTRITIONS

- Calories: 185 kcal
- Sugar: 3.9g
- Fat: 12.2g
- Carbohydrates: 20g
- Cholesterol: 0mg
- Protein: 3.5g

4. ORANGE CARROT KALE SALAD

 **PREPARATION TIME** 5'

 **COOK TIME** 12'

 **SERVING** 4

INGREDIENTS

- 8 cups kale, chopped
- 2 teaspoons olive oil
- 1 carrot, shredded
- ¼ teaspoon cumin, ground
- ⅛ teaspoon red chili flakes
- 1 onion, diced
- 2 garlic cloves, minced
- 1 red bell pepper, diced
- 1 cup fresh orange juice
- 1 teaspoon orange zest, grated
- Pepper to taste

DIRECTIONS

1. In a pan over medium heat warm the olive oil. Add onion to the pan and sauté for 2 minutes. Add bell pepper, garlic, orange juice, kale and stir well.
2. Reduce heat to medium-low and cook for another 5 minutes. Add in remaining ingredients and mix well.
3. Cover and cook for an additional 5 minutes. Serve immediately and enjoy!

NUTRITIONS

- Calories: 121 kcal
- Carbohydrates: 23.3g
- Fat: 1.9g
- Sugar: 5.2g
- Cholesterol: 0mg
- Protein: 5g

5. CREAMY PUMPKIN TOMATO SOUP

PREPARATION TIME
10'

COOK TIME
13'

SERVING
4

INGREDIENTS

- 2 cups pumpkin, diced
- ½ teaspoon paprika
- 1 ½ teaspoons curry powder
- ½ cup onion, chopped
- ½ teaspoon garlic, minced
- 2 cups vegetable broth, low-sodium
- 1 teaspoon extra-virgin olive oil
- ½ cup tomato, chopped

DIRECTIONS

1. In a pan add the olive oil, onion, garlic, and sauté over medium heat for 3 minutes. Add to pan remaining ingredients and bring to a boil.
2. Reduce the heat and cover, simmer for 10 minutes or until pumpkin is tender.
3. Using a blender puree the soup until smooth. Serve hot and enjoy!

NUTRITIONS

- Calories: 84 kcal
- Carbohydrates: 13.3g
- Fat: 2.4g
- Sugar: 5.6g
- Cholesterol: 0mg
- Protein: 4.3g

6. CREAMY CAULIFLOWER SOUP

PREPARATION TIME
10'

COOK TIME
19'

SERVING
4

INGREDIENTS

- 1 garlic clove, minced
- ½ head cauliflower, diced
- 1 small onion, diced
- 16 ounces vegetable broth
- ¼ tablespoon coconut oil
- 1 garlic clove, minced
- ½ teaspoon salt

DIRECTIONS

1. Heat the coconut oil in a pan over medium heat. Add the onion, garlic and sauté for 4 minutes. Add the vegetable broth and cauliflower. Bring to a boil.
2. Cover and simmer for 15 minutes. Season with salt.
3. Using blender puree the soup until smooth and creamy. Serve warm and enjoy!

NUTRITIONS

- Calories: 53 kcal
- Carbohydrates: 6.2g
- Sugar: 2.8g
- Cholesterol: 0mg
- Fat: 1.6g
- Protein: 4.1g

7. SPINACH GARLIC SALAD

PREPARATION TIME
10'

COOK TIME
2'

SERVING
2

INGREDIENTS

- 1 garlic clove, minced
- 8 ounces spinach, fresh, washed
- 1 green onion, chopped
- ¼ teaspoon sea salt
- 1 ½ teaspoons extra-virgin olive oil
- 1 ½ teaspoons soy sauce
- 2 teaspoons sesame seeds, toasted

DIRECTIONS

1. Boil four cups of water in a pan over high heat. Once the water is hot, blanch the spinach for 30 seconds.
2. Remove the spinach from heat and rinse in cold water. Squeeze out excess water from spinach.
3. In a bowl, add the green onion, garlic, oil, sesame seeds, soy sauce, and salt. Add the spinach and mix well. Serve fresh and enjoy!

NUTRITIONS

- Calories: 80 kcal
- Carbohydrates: 6.2 g
- Fat 5.4 g
- Sugar: 0.8 g
- Protein: 4.3 g
- Cholesterol: 0mg

8. ALMOND PEACH ARUGULA SALAD

PREPARATION TIME	COOK TIME	SERVING
15'	0	4

INGREDIENTS

- 6 cups baby arugula, washed, dried
- 1 tablespoon water
- ¼ teaspoon pepper
- ½ cup almonds, toasted, sliced
- 3 ripe peaches, pitted and sliced
- 1 tablespoon balsamic vinegar
- 1 tablespoon olive oil
- Pinch of salt

DIRECTIONS

1. In a mixing bowl, add the arugula, almonds, and peaches. Toss well.
2. In a small bowl, combine water, vinegar, salt and pour mixture over arugula mixture.
3. Season with salt and pepper. Serve fresh and enjoy!

NUTRITIONS

- Calories: 152 kcal
- Carbohydrates: 14.3g
- Fat: 9.9g
- Sugar: 11.6g
- Cholesterol: 0mg
- Protein: 4.3g

9. MUSHROOM FRITTATA

PREPARATION TIME
10'

COOK TIME
46'

SERVING
4

INGREDIENTS

- 6-ounces mushrooms, sliced
- 6 eggs, organic
- 1 cup leeks, sliced
- Sea salt

DIRECTIONS

1. Preheat your oven to 350°Fahrenheit. Spray a baking dish with cooking spray and set aside. Heat a pan over medium heat. Spray a pan with cooking spray.
2. Add the leeks and mushrooms to the pan and sauté for 6 minutes. Break eggs in a bowl, whisk well. Transfer the sautéed mushroom and leek mixture into the prepared baking dish.
3. Pour the eggs over the mushroom mixture. Bake in preheated oven for 40 minutes. Serve warm and enjoy!

NUTRITIONS

- Calories: 117 kcal
- Cholesterol: 246mg
- Sugar: 2.1g
- Fat: 6.8 g
- Carbohydrates: 5.1g
- Protein: 10g

10. ROASTED MUSHROOMS

PREPARATION TIME
10'

COOK TIME
30'

SERVING
2

INGREDIENTS

- 2 tablespoons olive oil
- 10 ounces mushrooms, quartered
- 2 garlic cloves, sliced
- 1 teaspoon thyme, chopped
- ¼ teaspoon pepper
- ¼ teaspoon sea salt

DIRECTIONS

1. Preheat your oven to 400°F. Spray a baking tray with cooking spray and set aside.
2. In a mixing bowl, combine the mushrooms, thyme, oil, salt, and pepper. Spread the mushrooms on a prepared baking sheet and bake in a preheated oven for 25 minutes.
3. Add garlic and mix well and cook for an additional 5 minutes. Serve and enjoy!

NUTRITIONS

- Calories: 157 kcal
- Carbohydrates: 6.1g
- Sugar: 2.5g
- Cholesterol: 0mg
- Fat: 14.5g
- Protein: 4.7g

11. COCONUT ALMOND EGG WRAPS

PREPARATION TIME

10'

COOK TIME

6'

SERVING

4

INGREDIENTS

- 5 eggs, organic
- 2 tablespoons almond meal
- 1 tablespoon coconut flour
- ¼ teaspoon sea salt

DIRECTIONS

1. In your blender add all the ingredients and blend until smooth. Heat a pan over medium-high heat that is non-stick. Pour two tablespoons of batter into a hot pan.
2. Cover and cook for 3 minutes. Flip over and cook for an additional 3 minutes. Serve hot and enjoy!

NUTRITIONS

- Calories: 111 kcal
- Fat: 7.5g
- Carbohydrates: 3.1g
- Sugar: 0.8g
- Cholesterol: 205mg
- Protein: 8.1g

12. BAKED EGG TOMATO

 **PREPARATION TIME**
5'

 **COOK TIME**
30'

 **SERVING**
2

INGREDIENTS

- 2 eggs, organic
- 2 large fresh tomatoes
- 1 teaspoon parsley, fresh, chopped
- Pepper and salt to taste

DIRECTIONS

1. Preheat your oven to 350°F. Cut off the top of the tomato and spoon out the innards.
2. Break an egg into each tomato, bake in a preheated oven for 30 minutes.
3. Season with parsley, pepper, and salt. Serve hot and enjoy!

NUTRITIONS

- Calories: 96 kcal
- Fat: 4.7g
- Carbohydrates: 7.5g
- Sugar: 5.1g
- Cholesterol: 164mg
- Protein: 7.2g

13. SPICY ASIAN STYLE TOFU

 **PREPARATION TIME** 5'

 **COOK TIME** 15'

 **SERVING** 4

INGREDIENTS

- 14 ounces tofu, extra-firm, cut into cubes
- 1 tablespoon ginger, fresh, chopped
- 1 green Chili, chopped
- 1 tablespoon coconut oil
- 1 teaspoon apple cider vinegar
- ¼ teaspoon cayenne powder
- 2 garlic cloves, chopped
- ½ teaspoon basil, dried
- 2 teaspoon sesame seeds
- 1 teaspoon garlic salt
- 1 tablespoon soy sauce
- 1 teaspoon Worcestershire sauce
- 2 tablespoons Sriracha chili sauce
- Pepper to taste
- 1 ½ tablespoons honey

DIRECTIONS

1. In a medium pan heat the coconut oil over medium heat. Add the green chili, garlic, and ginger; sauté for three minutes.
2. Add the tofu and sprinkle with some garlic salt. Sauté the tofu until it is lightly golden brown for about 15 minutes.
3. In a mixing bowl combine the honey, cayenne powder, soy sauce, sriracha chili sauce, and Worcestershire sauce.
4. Pour the honey mixture over the tofu and stir until well coated. Add the basil leaves and sesame seeds and stir. Serve hot and enjoy!

NUTRITIONS

- Calories: 154 kcal
- Fat: 8.4g
- Cholesterol: 0mg
- Sugar: 9.6g
- Carbohydrates: 13.2g
- Protein: 9.1g
-

14. GREEN BEANS WITH CHEESE

PREPARATION TIME
10'

COOK TIME
5'

SERVING
3

INGREDIENTS

- 1 lb. green beans
- ½ tablespoon butter
- ½ tablespoon coconut oil
- 1 ounce goat cheese
- 2 tablespoons walnuts, chopped
- 1 shallot, sliced
- Pepper and salt to taste

DIRECTIONS

1. Add salt and water to a pot and bring the water to a boil over medium heat. Add in the green beans and cook for 2 minutes, then drain and set aside.
2. Heat the coconut oil in a pan over medium heat. Add the shallots and cook until softened.
3. Add the butter, once the butter has melted add in the green beans and cook for an additional 3 minutes.
4. Transfer the beans into a bowl and toss with walnuts, cheese, pepper, and salt. Serve hot and enjoy!

NUTRITIONS

- Calories: 168 kcal
- Fat: 10.8g
- Carbohydrates: 13.8g
- Cholesterol: 15mg
- Sugar: 2.4g
- Protein: 7.2g

15. ZUCCHINI PATTIES

PREPARATION TIME
10'

COOK TIME
15'

SERVING
6

INGREDIENTS

- 1 egg, organic, beaten
- 1 ½ cups zucchini, shredded
- ¼ cup breadcrumbs
- ¼ cup cheddar cheese, shredded
- ¼ teaspoon salt
- ⅛ teaspoon pepper
- ¼ teaspoon basil
- ¼ teaspoon garlic powder

DIRECTIONS

1. Preheat your oven to 425°F. Spray a baking tray with cooking spray and set aside. Place your shredded zucchini on a paper towel and pat it dry.
2. Add the zucchini and remaining ingredients into a mixing bowl and blend well. Drop a tablespoon of mixture on the prepared baking tray and lightly flatten with a spoon.
3. Bake in preheated oven for 15 minutes or until golden brown. Serve warm and enjoy!

NUTRITIONS

- Calories: 52 kcal
- Fat: 2.6g
- Sugar: 0.9g
- Carbohydrates: 4.4g
- Cholesterol: 32mg
- Protein: 3.1g

16. CHILI CABBAGE WEDGES

PREPARATION TIME
5'

COOK TIME
20'

SERVING
4

INGREDIENTS

- 1 medium head cabbage
- 1 teaspoon chili powder
- Pepper and salt
- ¼ cup olive oil

DIRECTIONS

1. Start by preheating the oven to 400°F.
2. Divide the cabbage into wedges then spread them out onto a baking sheet.
3. Add the chili powder, pepper, and salt to season. Sprinkle the olive oil on the cabbage and mix properly.
4. Put them in the oven. Bake for about 20 minutes or until the wedges turn to a nice color.
5. Transfer to four serving bowls. Allow cooling for a few minutes before serving.

NUTRITIONS

- Calories: 108 kcal
- Total Fat: 10g
- Fiber: 3g
- Net Carbs: 3g
- Protein: 1.5g

17. CAULIFLOWER, LEEKS AND BROCCOLI

PREPARATION TIME
5'

COOK TIME
15'

SERVING
4

INGREDIENTS

- 8 ounces cauliflower, chopped into bite-sized pieces
- 3 ounces leeks, chopped into bite-sized pieces
- 1 pound broccoli, chopped into bite-sized pieces
- 3 ounces butter
- 5 ounces shredded cheese
- ½ cup fresh thyme
- Pepper and salt to taste
- 4 tablespoons sour cream

DIRECTIONS

1. In a skillet over medium-high heat, add butter and heat to melt. Add the leeks, broccoli and cauliflower. Fry the vegetables until they become golden brown.
2. Add the cheese, thyme and sour cream. Stir well until the cheese melts. Add pepper and salt for seasoning.
3. Transfer them to a platter. Allow cooling for a few minutes before serving

NUTRITIONS

- Calories: 368 kcal
- Total Fat: 32g
- Fiber: 5.4g
- Net Carbs: 9.3g
- Protein: 14.2g

18. ROASTED GREEN BEANS WITH PARMESAN

PREPARATION TIME	COOK TIME	SERVING
10'	20'	4

INGREDIENTS

- 1 pound fresh green beans
- 1 egg
- ½ teaspoon salt
- ¼ teaspoon pepper
- 2 tablespoons olive oil
- 1 teaspoon onion powder
- 1 ounce grated Parmesan cheese

DIRECTIONS

1. Start by preheating the oven to 400°F.
2. In a bowl, whisk the egg, salt, pepper, oil, and onion powder.
3. Add the green beans, and then toss to coat well.
4. Drain the excess liquid, and then arrange the green beans on a baking sheet lined with parchment paper. Sprinkle with Parmesan cheese.
5. Bake in the oven for about 20 minutes until the beans change to a nice color.
6. Transfer to four serving plates. Allow cooling for a few minutes before serving.

NUTRITIONS

- Calories: 143 kcal
- Total Fat: 11g
- Fiber: 2.5g
- Net Carbs: 5.8g
- Protein: 6.2g
-

8. POULTRY AND MEAT RECIPES

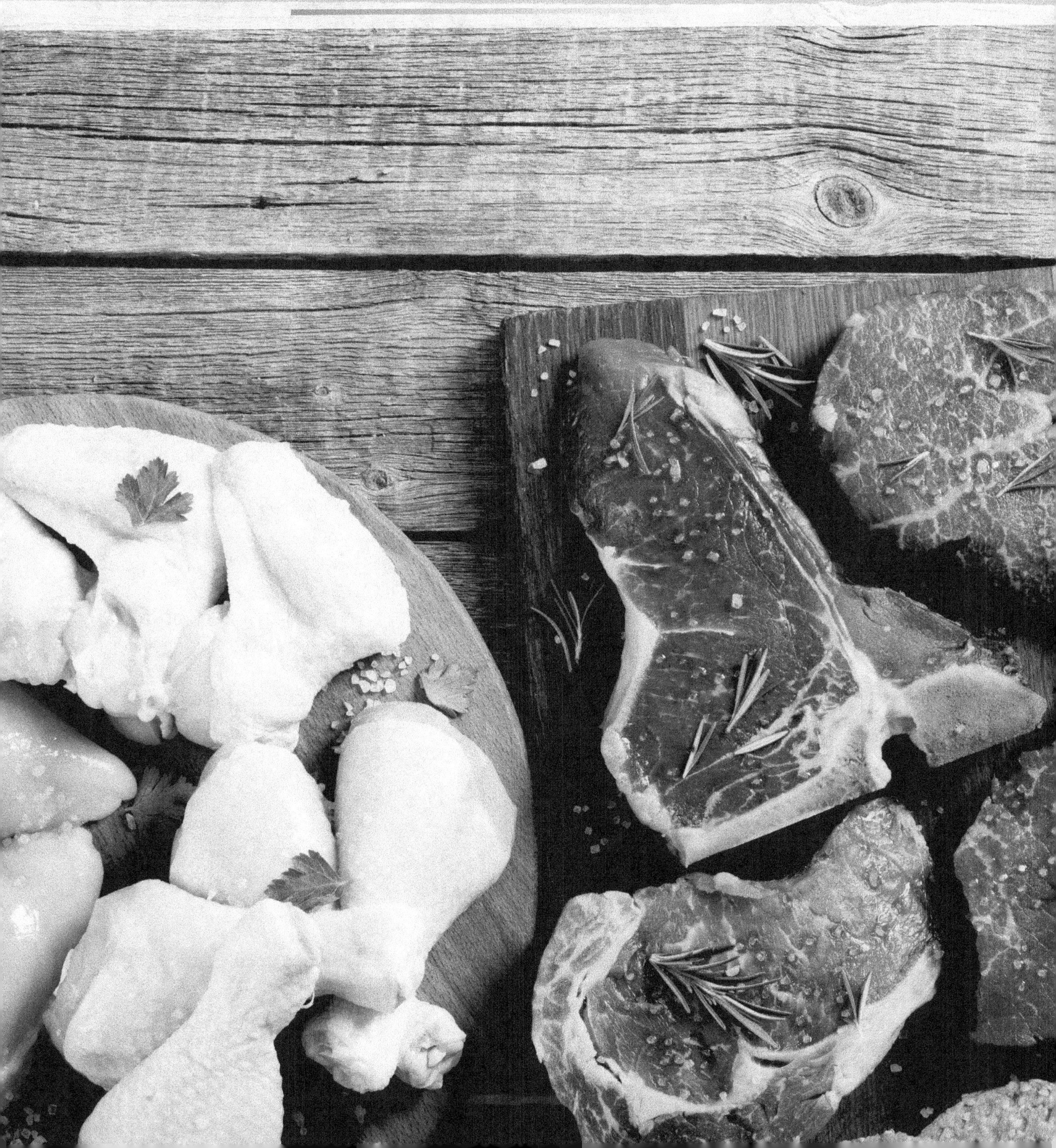

1. TURKEY MEATLOAF

PREPARATION TIME
10'

COOK TIME
1 H 5'

SERVING
6

INGREDIENTS

- 2 tablespoons extra-virgin olive oil
- 2 teaspoons minced garlic
- ½ onion, chopped
- ½ cup ground almonds
- ½ cup heavy whipping cream
- 1 large egg, beaten
- 1 pound ground turkey
- 1 tablespoon chopped fresh parsley
- 8 ounces (227 g) turkey sausage meat
- Salt and freshly ground black pepper, to taste

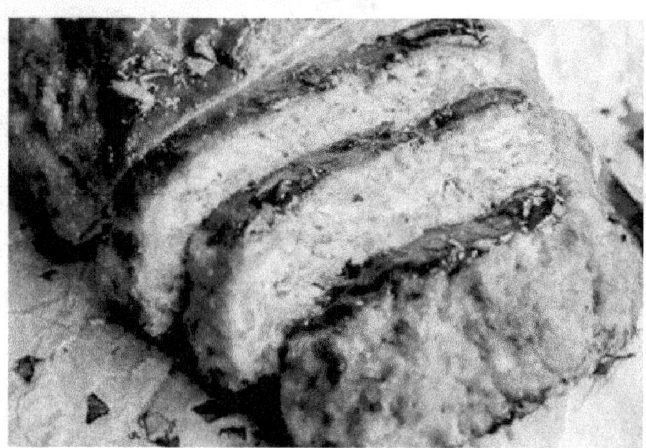

DIRECTIONS

1. Preheat the oven to 350°F (180°C).
2. Warm the olive oil in a nonstick skillet over medium-high heat.
3. Add the garlic and onion to the skillet and sauté for 3 minutes or until the onion is translucent.
4. Transfer the cooked garlic and onion to a large bowl, and then add the remaining ingredients. Stir to mix well.
5. Pour the mixture into a meatloaf pan, and press with a spatula.
6. Bake in the preheated oven for 1 hour until the meatloaf is golden brown.
7. Remove the meatloaf from the oven. Allow to cool for 10 minutes and serve.

NUTRITIONS

- Calories: 356 kcal
- Total Fat: 28.1g
- Total Carbs: 5.9g
- Fiber: 3.1g
- Net Carbs: 2.8g
- Protein: 20.8g

KETO DIET COOKBOOK FOR WOMEN OVER 50

2. TURKEY, BABY SPINACH, AND ZUCCHINI FRITTATA

PREPARATION TIME
15'

COOK TIME
30'

SERVING
4

INGREDIENTS

- 6 large eggs, beaten
- ½ cup heavy whipping cream
- Salt and freshly ground black pepper, to taste
- 3 tablespoons extra-virgin olive oil
- 8 ounces (227 g) turkey breast, diced
- 2 teaspoons garlic, minced
- ½ onion, chopped
- 2 yellow zucchini, shredded
- 2 cups fresh baby spinach leaves

DIRECTIONS

1. Preheat the oven to 375°F (190°C).
2. Combine the beaten eggs and cream in a bowl. Sprinkle it with salt and black pepper. Set aside until ready to use.
3. Warm the olive oil in an oven-safe skillet over medium-high heat.
4. Add the turkey breast to the skillet and cook for 6 to 8 minutes until an instant-read thermometer inserted in the thickest part of the turkey registers at least 150°F (66°C). Flip over the turkey breast halfway through. Set aside.
5. Add the garlic and onion to the skillet and sauté for 3 minutes or until the onion is translucent.
6. Add the zucchini and spinach to the skillet and sauté for 4 minutes or until fork-tender.
7. Add the cooked turkey back to the skillet and stir to combine well.
8. To make the frittata: pour the egg mixture over the turkey and cook for 3 minutes or until the eggs are set and they no longer jiggle.
9. Place the oven-safe skillet in the preheated oven and bake for 20 minutes. Cut a small slit in the center, if raw eggs run into the cut, continue baking for another few minutes.

NUTRITIONS

- Calories: 434 kcal
- Total Fat: 33.3g
- Total Carbs: 6.7g
- Fiber: 2.1g
- Net Carbs: 4.6g
- Protein: 27.1g

3. CHICKEN AND AVOCADO WRAPPED LETTUCE

 **PREPARATION TIME**
10'

 **COOK TIME**
5'

 **SERVING**
4

INGREDIENTS

- 2 tablespoons extra-virgin olive oil
- 6 ounces (170 g) chicken breasts, chopped
- Salt and freshly ground black pepper, to taste
- ½ avocado, peeled, pitted, and mashed
- 2 teaspoons thyme, fresh and chopped
- ⅓ cup creamy mayonnaise, keto-friendly
- 1 teaspoon freshly squeezed lemon juice
- 8 large lettuce leaves
- ¼ cup walnuts, chopped

DIRECTIONS

1. Warm the olive oil in an oven-safe skillet over medium-high heat.
2. Put the chopped chicken breasts in the skillet, and sprinkle with salt and black pepper. Sauté for 5 minutes or until well browned. Set aside.
3. Combine the mashed avocado, thyme, mayo, and lemon juice in a bowl, and then add the cooked chicken. Toss to mix well.
4. Divide and arrange the mixture on the lettuce leaves, then top it with walnuts before serving.

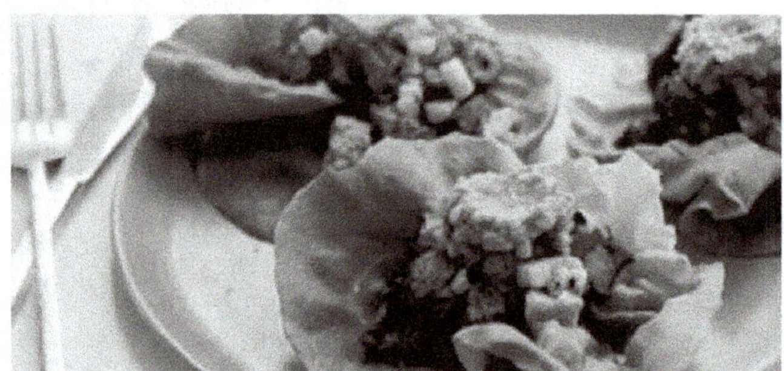

NUTRITIONS

- Calories: 253 kcal
- Total Fat: 20.1g
- Carbs: 5.9g
- Protein: 12.1g

4. SPICY CHICKEN BREASTS

PREPARATION TIME
10'

COOK TIME
25'

SERVING
4

INGREDIENTS

- 2 tablespoons olive oil
- 4 chicken breasts, skin on
- Salt and freshly ground black pepper, to taste
- ½ cup sweet onion, chopped
- ½ cup heavy whipping cream
- 2 teaspoons smoked paprika
- 2 cups sour cream
- 2 tablespoons parsley, chopped

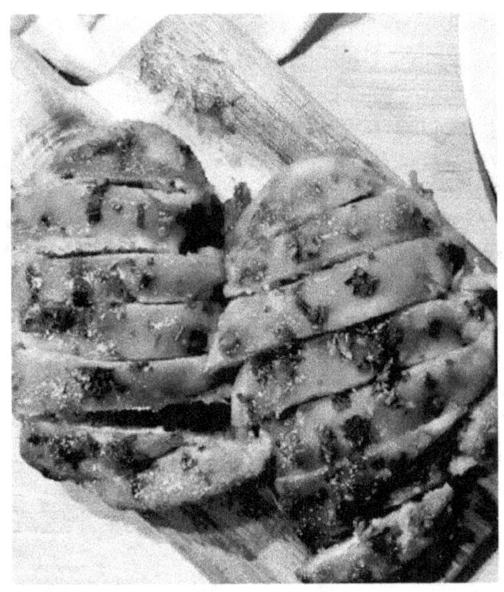

DIRECTIONS

1. Heat the olive oil in a nonstick skillet over medium-high heat until shimmering.
2. Put the chicken breasts in the skillet, skin side down, and sprinkle with salt and black pepper. Sear for 5 minutes per side or until lightly browned. Flip the chicken breasts halfway through the cooking time. Set aside.
3. Add the onion to the skillet and sauté for 4 minutes or until translucent.
4. Mix in the cream and paprika, and then bring the mixture to a simmer.
5. Put the chicken back in the skillet, and simmer for an additional 5 minutes.
6. Remove the chicken breasts from the skillet. Spread the sour cream and parsley on top before serving.

NUTRITIONS

- Calories: 392 kcal
- Total Fat: 30.1g
- Carbs: 3.8g
- Protein: 25.1g

5. CHICKEN CAPRESE

PREPARATION TIME
15'

COOK TIME
40'

SERVING
4

INGREDIENTS

- ¼ cup extra-virgin olive oil, divided
- 4 (4-ounce / 113-g) boneless chicken breasts
- Salt and freshly ground black pepper, to taste
- 1 tablespoon minced garlic
- 1 (28-ounce/794-g) can diced tomatoes
- Red pepper flakes, to taste
- 2 tablespoons chopped fresh basil
- 4 ounces (113 g) shredded Mozzarella cheese

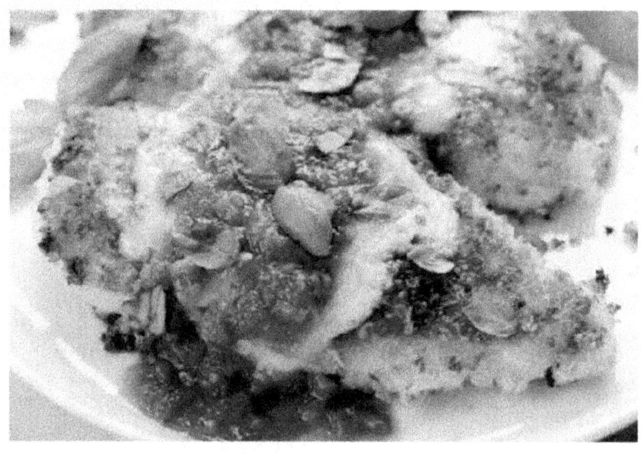

DIRECTIONS

1. Preheat the oven to 400°F (205°C).
2. Heat 2 tablespoons of the olive oil in an oven-safe skillet over medium-high heat until shimmering.
3. Put the chicken breasts in the skillet, and sprinkle with salt and black pepper. Sear for 5 minutes per side or until lightly browned. Flip the chicken breasts halfway through the cooking time. Set aside.
4. To make the sauce: heat the remaining olive oil in the skillet over medium-high heat. Sauté the garlic in the skillet for 2 minutes until fragrant, then mix in the tomatoes, red pepper flakes, and basil. Sauté for another 5 minutes until well combined and has a thick consistency.
5. Put the chicken breasts back to the skillet, and spoon the sauce over to coat them, and then scatter the mozzarella cheese over.
6. Put the skillet lid on and bake in the preheated oven for 25 minutes or until an instant-read thermometer inserted in the thickest part of the chicken breasts registers at least 165°F (74°C).
7. Remove the chicken breasts and sauce from the oven and serve hot.

NUTRITIONS

- Calories: 433 kcal
- Total Fat: 32.2g
- Total Carbs: 8.9g
- Fiber: 3.1g
- Net Carbs: 5.8g
- Protein: 29.1g

6. RICOTTA, PROSCIUTTO, AND SPINACH CHICKEN ROLLATINI

PREPARATION TIME
15'

COOK TIME
35'

SERVING
4

INGREDIENTS

- 4 ounces (113 g) ricotta cheese
- 4 (3-ounce/85-g) boneless skinless chicken breasts, pounded to about ⅓-inch thick
- 4 (1-ounce/28-g) slices prosciutto
- 1 cup fresh spinach
- 2 eggs
- ½ cup almond flour
- ½ cup grated parmesan cheese
- ¼ cup extra-virgin olive oil
- Salt and freshly ground black pepper, to taste

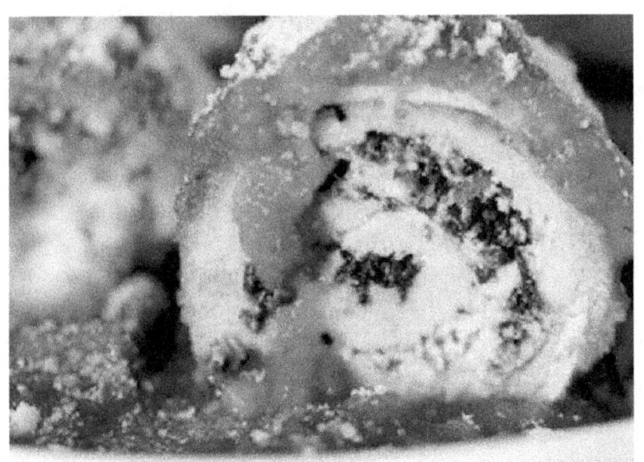

DIRECTIONS

1. Preheat the oven to 400°F (205°C).
2. To make the rollatini: On a clean work surface, put 1 ounce (28 g) of ricotta cheese on the center of a chicken breast, then top the ricotta cheese with a slice of prosciutto, and ¼ cup of the spinach. Repeat with the remaining chicken breasts, ricotta cheese, prosciutto, and spinach.
3. Roll up the chicken breasts to wrap the filling, then secure with two toothpicks. Set aside.
4. Whisk the eggs in a bowl. Combine the almond flour and parmesan cheese in another bowl.
5. Dredge the chicken rollatini in the whisked eggs, and then dunk in the almond flour mixture to coat well.
6. Heat the olive oil in an oven-safe skillet over medium heat until shimmering.
7. Arrange the chicken rollatini in the skillet, seam side down, and sprinkle with salt and black pepper. Fry for 10 minutes or until well browned. Gently flip them halfway through the cooking time.
8. Bake the chicken rollatini in the preheated oven for 25 minutes or until an instant-read thermometer inserted in the thickest part of the chicken breasts registers at least 165°F (74°C).
9. Transfer the chicken rollatini onto four plates. Remove the toothpicks and serve warm.

NUTRITIONS

- Calories: 439 kcal
- Total Fat: 30.1g
- Total Carbs: 1.9g
- Fiber: 0g
- Net Carbs: 1.9g
- Protein: 40.2g

PREPARATION TIME	COOK TIME	SERVING
10'	45'	6T

INGREDIENTS

- 3 tablespoons extra-virgin olive oil, divided
- ½ pound (227 g) Italian sausage, sweet or hot
- 1 pound (454 g) boneless chicken thighs
- Salt and freshly ground black pepper, to taste
- 1 pepper, chopped
- 1 tablespoon minced garlic
- ¼ cup dry white wine
- 1 cup chicken stock
- 2 tablespoons chopped fresh parsley

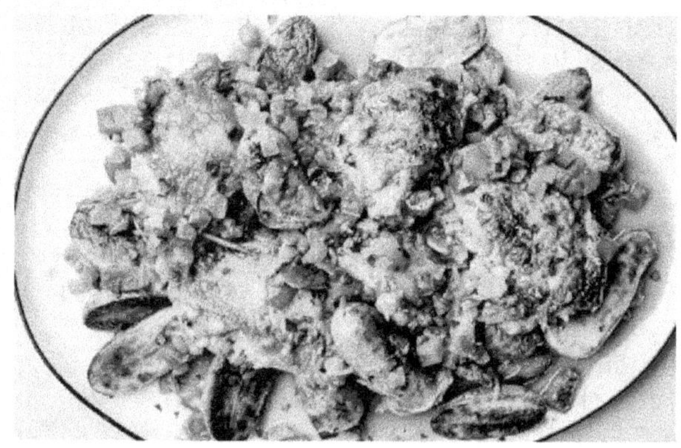

DIRECTIONS

1. Preheat the oven to 425°F (220°C).
2. Heat 2 tablespoons of the olive oil in an oven-safe skillet over medium-high heat until shimmering.
3. Put the sausage and chicken thighs in the skillet, and sprinkle with salt and black pepper. Sear for 5 minutes per side or until lightly browned. Flip them halfway through the cooking time. Set aside.
4. Arrange the skillet in the preheated oven and bake for 25 minutes or until an instant-read thermometer inserted in the thickest part of the chicken breasts registers at least 165°F (74°C). Transfer them to a plate. Set aside.
5. Heat the remaining olive oil in the skillet over medium-high heat until shimmering.
6. Sauté the pepper and garlic in the skillet for 3 minutes until fragrant, then pour the dry white wine over for deglazing.
7. Pour the chicken stock into the skillet, and then bring them to a boil. Turn down the heat to low and simmer for 6 minutes until it reduces to half.
8. Put the sausage and chicken back in the skillet, and toss to coat well. Transfer them to a plate, and spread the parsley on top before serving.

NUTRITIONS

- Calories: 372 kcal
- Total Fat: 30.1g
- Total Carbs: 2.9g
- Fiber: 0g
- Net Carbs: 2.9g
- Protein: 19.1g

8. CHICKEN THIGH AND TOMATO BRAISE

PREPARATION TIME
10'

COOK TIME
4 HOURS

SERVING
4T

INGREDIENTS

- ¼ cup olive oil, divided
- 4 (4-ounce/113-g) boneless chicken thighs
- Salt and freshly ground black pepper, to taste
- ½ cup chicken stock
- 4 ounces (113 g) julienned oil-packed sun-dried tomatoes
- 1 (28-ounce/794-g) can sodium-free diced tomatoes
- 2 tablespoons dried oregano
- 2 tablespoons minced garlic
- Red pepper flakes, to taste
- 2 tablespoons chopped fresh parsley

DIRECTIONS

1. Coat the inside of the slow cooker with 1 tablespoon of olive oil.
2. Heat the remaining olive oil in a nonstick skillet over medium-high heat, then put the chicken thighs in the skillet and sprinkle salt and black pepper to season.
3. Sear the chicken thighs for 10 minutes or until well browned. Flip them halfway through the cooking time.
4. Put the chicken thighs, stock, tomatoes, oregano, garlic, and red pepper flakes into the slow cooker. Stir to coat the chicken thighs well.
5. Put the slow cooker lid on and cook on high setting for 4 hours until an instant-read thermometer inserted in the thickest part of the chicken thighs registers at least 165°F (74°C).
6. Transfer the chicken thighs to four plates. Pour the sauce which remains in the slow cooker over the chicken thighs and top with fresh parsley before serving warm.

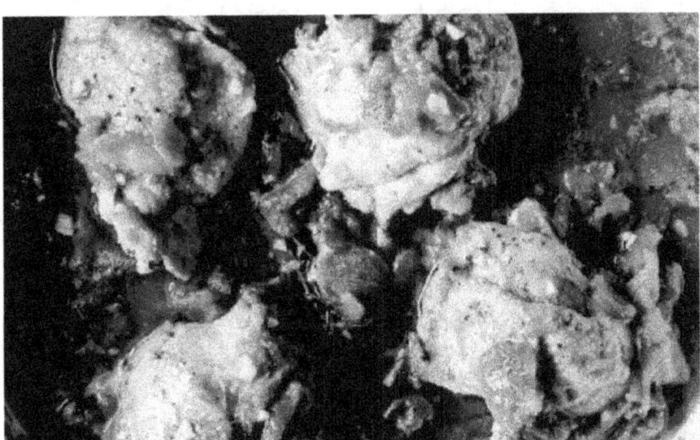

NUTRITIONS

- Calories: 469 kcal
- Total Fat: 36.1g
- Total Carbs: 13.7g
- Fiber: 7.3g
- Net Carbs: 6.4g
- Protein: 24.2g

9. TOMATO AND EGGPLANT WITH RICH CHICKEN THIGHS

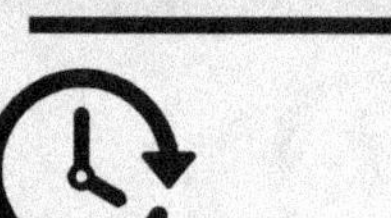

PREPARATION TIME
10'

COOK TIME
20'

SERVING
4

INGREDIENTS

- 2 tablespoons butter
- 1 pound (454 g) chicken thighs
- Salt and freshly ground black pepper, to taste
- 2 garlic cloves, minced
- 1 (14-ounce/397-g) can whole tomatoes
- 1 eggplant, diced
- 10 fresh basil leaves, chopped, plus more for garnish

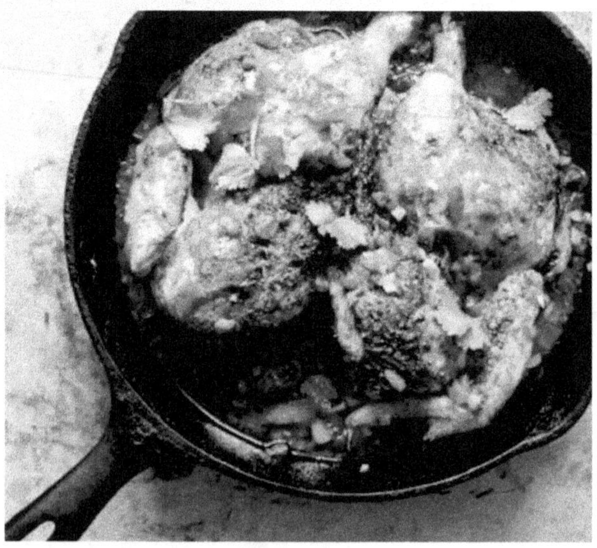

DIRECTIONS

1. Put the butter in a nonstick skillet, melt over medium heat.
2. Put the chicken thighs in the skillet, and sprinkle with salt and black pepper. Fry for 8 minutes or until well browned. Flip the chicken thighs halfway through the cooking time.
3. Transfer the chicken thighs to a plate, and then add the garlic to the skillet. Sauté in the remaining butter for 2 minutes or until fragrant.
4. Add the tomatoes to the skillet and sauté for 8 minutes or until lightly softened.
5. Add the eggplant and basil to the skillet, and cook for 4 more minutes until tender. Sprinkle salt and black pepper to season.
6. Put the chicken thighs back to the skillet, and spoon the sauce in the skillet over the chicken thighs to coat well.
7. Put the lid on and simmer for 3 minutes or until the internal temperature of the chicken thighs reach at least 165°F (74°C).
8. Transfer the chicken and the sauce to a large plate and serve with more basil on top.

NUTRITIONS

- Calories: 469 kcal
- Total Fat: 39.7g
- Carbs: 1.9g
- Protein: 26.1g

KETO DIET COOKBOOK FOR WOMEN OVER 50

10. JERK PORK

PREPARATION TIME	COOK TIME	SERVING
15'	20'	6

INGREDIENTS

Jerk seasoning:
- ⅛ teaspoon cayenne pepper
- ¼ teaspoon salt
- ¼ teaspoon freshly ground black pepper
- ½ tablespoon dried thyme
- ½ tablespoon garlic powder
- ½ tablespoon ground allspice
- 1 teaspoon ground cinnamon
- 1 tablespoon granulated erythritol
- 1 (1-pound/454-g) pork tenderloin, cut into 1-inch rounds
- ¼ cup extra-virgin olive oil
- 2 tablespoons chopped fresh cilantro, for garnish
- ½ cup sour cream

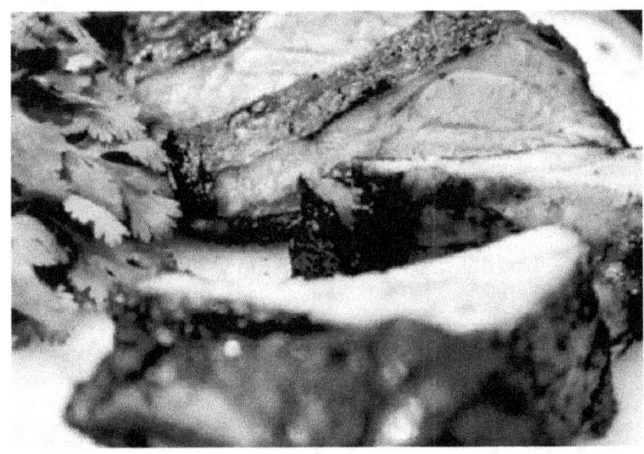

DIRECTIONS

1. Combine the ingredients for the seasoning in a bowl. Stir to mix well.
2. Put the pork rounds in the bowl of seasoning mixture. Toss to coat well.
3. Pour the olive oil into a nonstick skillet, and heat over medium-high heat.
4. Arrange the pork in a single layer in the skillet and fry for 20 minutes or until an instant-read thermometer inserted in the center of the pork registers at least 145°F (63°C). Flip the pork around halfway through the cooking time. You may need to work in batches to avoid overcrowding.
5. Transfer the pork rounds onto a large platter, and top with cilantro and sour cream, then serve warm.

NUTRITIONS

- Calories: 289 kcal
- Total Fat: 23.2g
- Total Carbs: 2.8g
- Fiber: 0.9g
- Net Carbs: 1.9g
- Protein: 17.2g

11. HOT PORK AND BELL PEPPER IN LETTUCE

PREPARATION TIME
15'

COOK TIME
20'

SERVING
4

INGREDIENTS

Sauce:
- 1 tablespoon fish sauce
- 1 tablespoon rice vinegar
- 1 tablespoon almond flour
- 1 teaspoon coconut aminos
- 1 tablespoon granulated erythritol
- 2 tablespoons coconut oil

Pork filling:
- 2 tablespoons sesame oil, divided
- 1 pound (454 g) ground pork
- 1 teaspoon fresh ginger, peeled and grated
- 1 teaspoon garlic, minced
- 1 red bell pepper, deseeded and thinly sliced
- 1 scallion, white and green parts, thinly sliced
- 8 large romaine or Boston lettuce leaves

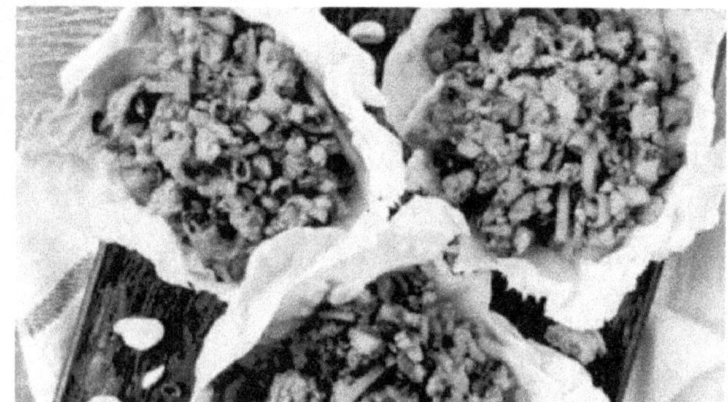

DIRECTIONS

1. To make the sauce: Combine the ingredients for the sauce in a bowl. Set aside until ready to use.
2. To make the pork filling: In a nonstick skillet, warm a tablespoon of sesame oil over medium-high heat.
3. Add and sauté the ground pork for 8 minutes or until lightly browned, then pour the sauce over and keep cooking for 4 more minutes or until the sauce has lightly thickened.
4. Transfer the pork onto a platter and set aside until ready to use.
5. Clean the skillet with paper towels, and then warm the remaining sesame oil over medium-high heat.
6. Add and sauté the ginger and garlic for 3 minutes or until fragrant.
7. Add and sauté the sliced bell pepper and scallion for an additional 5 minutes or until fork-tender.
8. Lower the heat, and move the pork back to the skillet. Stir to combine well.
9. Divide and arrange the pork filling over four lettuce leaves and serve hot.

NUTRITIONS

- Calories: 385 kcal
- Total Fat: 31.1g
- Total Carbs: 5.8g
- Fiber: 1.9g
- Net Carbs: 3.9g
- Protein: 20.1g

12. ITALIAN SAUSAGE, ZUCCHINI, EGGPLANT, AND TOMATO RATATOUILLE

PREPARATION TIME
15'

COOK TIME
45'

SERVING
4

INGREDIENTS

- 3 tablespoons extra-virgin olive oil
- 1 pound (454 g) Italian sausage meat, sweet or hot
- 2 zucchini, diced
- 1 red bell pepper, diced
- ½ eggplant, cut into ½-inch cubes
- 1 tablespoon garlic, minced
- ½ red onion, chopped
- 1 tablespoon balsamic vinegar
- 1 (15-ounce/425-g) can low-sodium tomatoes, diced
- 1 tablespoon fresh basil, chopped
- Red pepper flakes, to taste
- 2 teaspoons chopped fresh oregano, for garnish
- Salt and freshly ground black pepper, to taste

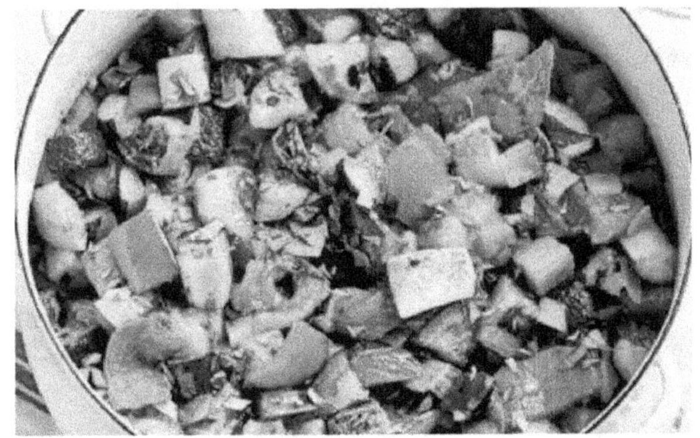

DIRECTIONS

1. Add the olive oil in a stock pot, and warm over medium-high heat, then add and sauté the Italian sausage meat for 7 minutes or until lightly browned.
2. Add the zucchini, bell pepper, eggplant, garlic, and onion to the pot and sauté for 10 minutes or until tender.
3. Fold in the balsamic vinegar, tomatoes, basil, and red pepper flakes. Stir to combine well, and then bring it to a boil.
4. Turn down the heat to low. Simmer the mixture for 25 minutes or until the vegetables are entirely softened.
5. Sprinkle it with oregano, salt, and black pepper. Stir to mix well, then serve warm.

NUTRITIONS

- Calories: 431 kcal
- Total Fat: 33.2g
- Total Carbs: 11.8g
- Fiber: 4.2g
- Net Carbs: 7.6g
- Protein: 21.2g

13. BACON, BEEF, AND PECAN PATTIES

PREPARATION TIME
10'

COOK TIME
15'

SERVING
8

INGREDIENTS

- ¼ cup chopped onion
- ¼ cup ground pecans
- 1 large egg
- 2 ounces (57 g) cheddar cheese, diced
- 8 ounces (227 g) bacon, chopped
- 1 pound (454 g) grass-fed ground beef
- Salt and freshly ground black pepper, to taste
- 1 tablespoon extra-virgin olive oil

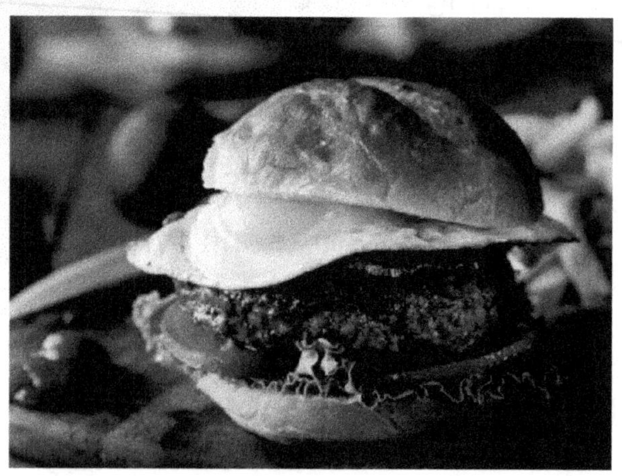

DIRECTIONS

1. Preheat the oven to 450°F (235°C). Line a baking sheet with parchment paper.
2. Whisk together all the ingredients, except for the olive oil, in a bowl.
3. Grease your hands with olive oil, and shape the mixture into 8 patties with your hands.
4. Arrange the patties on the baking sheet and bake in the preheated oven for 20 minutes or until a meat thermometer inserted in the center of the patties reads at least 165°F (74°C). Flip the patties halfway through the cooking time.
5. Remove the cooked patties from the oven and serve warm.

NUTRITIONS

- Calories: 318 kcal
- Total Fat: 27.2g
- Total Carbs: 1.1g
- Fiber: 1.1g
- Net Carbs: 0g
- Protein: 18.1g

14. LEMONY ANCHOVY BUTTER WITH STEAKS

PREPARATION TIME	COOK TIME	SERVING
15'	10'	4

INGREDIENTS

Anchovy butter:
- 4 anchovies packed in oil, drained and minced
- ½ teaspoon freshly squeezed lemon juice
- ¼ cup unsalted butter, at room temperature
- 1 teaspoon minced garlic
- 4 (4-ounce/113-g) rib-eye steaks
- Salt and freshly ground black pepper, to taste

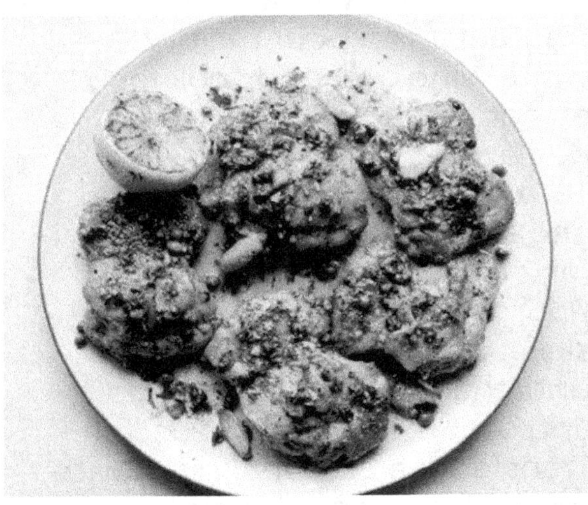

DIRECTIONS

1. To make the anchovy butter: combine the anchovies, lemon juice, butter, and garlic in a bowl. Stir to mix well, and then arrange the bowl into the refrigerator to chill until ready to use.
2. Preheat the grill to medium-high heat.
3. Rub the steaks with salt and black pepper on a clean work surface.
4. Arrange the seasoned steaks on the grill grates and grill for 10 minutes or until medium-rare. Flip the steaks halfway through the cooking time.
5. Allow the steaks to cool for 10 minutes. Transfer the steaks onto four plates, and spread the anchovy butter on top, then serve warm.

NUTRITIONS

- Calories: 447
- Total Fat: 38.1g
- Total Carbs: 0g
- Fiber: 0g
- Net Carbs: 0g
- Protein: 26.1g

15. ZUCCHINI CARBONARA

 **PREPARATION TIME**
10'

 **COOK TIME**
15'

 **SERVING**
6

INGREDIENTS

- 8 chopped bacon slices
- 2 large eggs
- 4 large egg yolks
- ½ cup grated parmesan cheese, divided
- ½ cup heavy whipping cream
- 2 tablespoons chopped fresh basil
- 2 tablespoons chopped fresh parsley
- Salt and freshly ground black pepper, to taste
- 1 tablespoon minced garlic
- ½ cup dry white wine
- 4 medium zucchini, spiralized

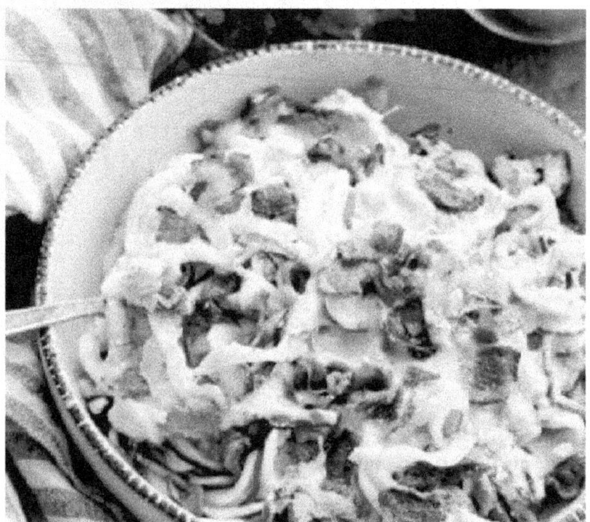

DIRECTIONS

1. In a nonstick skillet, cook the bacon for 6 minutes or until it curls and buckle. Flip the bacon halfway through the cooking time.
2. Meanwhile, whisk together the eggs, egg yolks, ¼ cup of parmesan cheese, cream, basil, parsley, salt, and black pepper in a large bowl. Set aside.
3. Add the garlic to the skillet and sauté for 3 minutes until fragrant, then pour the dry white wine over and cook for an additional 2 minutes for deglazing.
4. Turn down the heat to low, add and sauté the spiralized zucchini for 2 minutes.
5. Pour the egg mixture into the skillet and toss for 4 minutes or until the mixture is thickened and coat the spiralized zucchini.
6. Transfer to a platter and top with remaining cheese before serving.

NUTRITIONS

- Calories: 332 kcal
- Total Fat: 26.2g
- Total Carbs: 6.9g
- Fiber: 2.1g
- Net Carbs: 4.8g
- Protein: 19.1g

18. MUSHROOM, SPINACH, AND ONION STUFFED MEATLOAF

PREPARATION TIME	COOK TIME	SERVING
20'	1 HOUR	8

INGREDIENTS

- 3 tablespoons extra-virgin olive oil
- 17 ounces (482 g) ground beef
- 2 teaspoons ground cumin
- 2 garlic cloves, granulated
- Salt and freshly ground black pepper, to taste
- 6 slices Cheddar cheese
- ¼ cup mushrooms, diced
- ½ cup spinach
- ¼ cup onions, diced
- ¼ cup green onions, diced

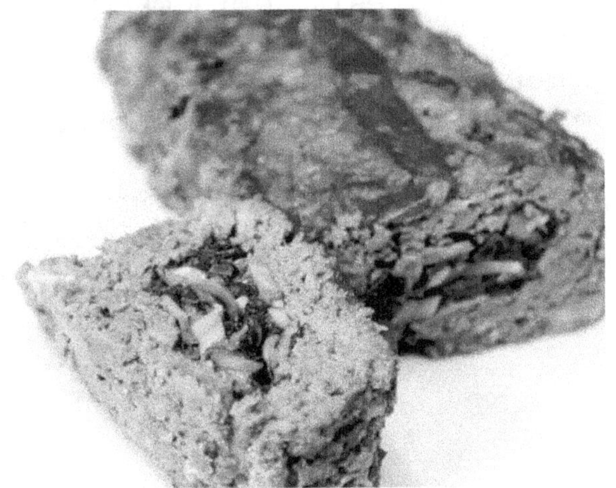

DIRECTIONS

1. Preheat the oven to 350°F (180°C). Coat a meatloaf pan with olive oil.
2. Combine 1 pound (454 g) ground beef, cumin, garlic, salt, and black pepper in a large bowl. Pour the mixture into the meatloaf pan.
3. Make a well in the center of the beef mixture, and then scatter the cheese on the bottom of the well. Put the mushrooms, spinach, and onions in the well, then cover them with the remaining 1 ounce (28 g) ground beef.
4. Place the meatloaf pan into the preheated oven and bake for 1 hour until cooked through.
5. Remove the meatloaf from the oven and slice to serve.

NUTRITIONS

- Calories: 254 kcal
- Total Fat: 20.2g
- Carbs: 1.4g
- Protein: 15.3g

17. ITALIAN FLAVOR HERBED PORK CHOPS

PREPARATION TIME
10'

COOK TIME
20'

SERVING
4T

INGREDIENTS

- 2 tablespoons melted butter, plus more for coating
- 2 tablespoons Italian seasoning
- 2 tablespoons olive oil
- Salt and freshly ground black pepper, to taste (if there isn't salt or pepper in the Italian seasoning)
- 4 pork chops, boneless
- 2 tablespoons fresh Italian leaf parsley, chopped

DIRECTIONS

1. Preheat the oven to 350°F (180°C). Grease a baking dish with melted butter.
2. Combine the Italian seasoning, butter, olive oil, salt, and black pepper in a large bowl. Dredge each pork chop into the bowl to coat well.
3. Arrange the pork chops onto the baking dish, and spread the fresh parsley on top of each chop.
4. Bake in the preheated oven for 20 minutes or until cooked through and an instant-read thermometer inserted in the middle of the pork chops register at least 145°F (63°C).
5. Transfer the pork chops from the oven and serve warm.

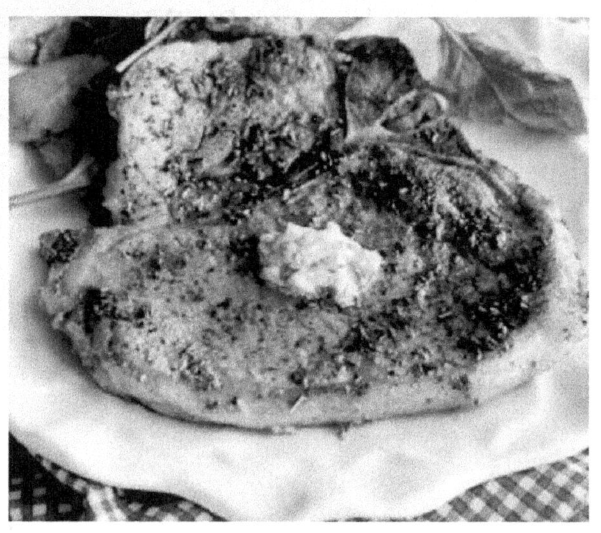

NUTRITIONS

- Calories: 335 kcal
- Total Fat: 23.4g
- Carbs: 0g
- Protein: 30.9g

PREPARATION TIME
10'

COOK TIME
4 HOURS

SERVING
8

INGREDIENTS

- 3 tablespoons olive oil, plus more for greasing the slow cooker
- 5 garlic cloves, finely chopped
- 1 onion, finely chopped
- 2 pounds (907 g) beef, minced
- 2 teaspoons dried mixed herbs (oregano, rosemary, thyme)
- 4 tomatoes, chopped
- Salt and freshly ground black pepper, to taste
- 1 large eggplant, cut into round slices crosswise
- 2 large zucchinis, cut into slices lengthwise
- 2 cups baby spinach leaves
- 1 cup ricotta cheese
- 1 cup Mozzarella cheese, grated
- 2 cups Cheddar cheese, grated

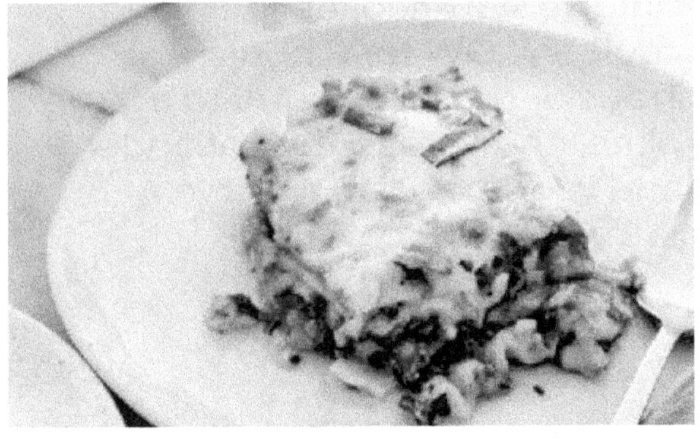

DIRECTIONS

1. Warm the olive oil in a nonstick skillet over medium-high heat.
2. Add and sauté the garlic and onions for 3 minutes or until the onions are translucent.
3. Add and sauté the beef for 3 more minutes until lightly browned.
4. Add the dried mixed herbs and tomatoes over the beef, and season with salt and black pepper. Sauté for 5 minutes to combine well.
5. Grease the slow cooker with olive oil.
6. To make the lasagna: Spread a layer of beef mixture on the bottom of the slow cooker, and top the beef mixture with a layer of eggplant slices, then spread another layer of beef mixture, and then put on a layer of zucchini slices, after that, top the zucchini slices with a layer of beef mixture, then spread a layer of baby spinach leaves, and finally, a layer of beef mixture.
7. Combine all the cheeses, salt, and black pepper in a large bowl. Scatter the cheese mixture over the lasagna.
8. Put the slow cooker lid on and bake on a high setting for 4 hours.
9. Remove the hot lasagna from the slow cooker and slice to serve.

NUTRITIONS

- Calories: 397 kcal
- Total Fat: 22.0g
- Carbs: 10.5g
- Protein: 40.8g

19. LAMB AND TOMATO CURRY

 **PREPARATION TIME**
10'

 **COOK TIME**
8 HOURS

 **SERVING**
8

INGREDIENTS

- 3 tablespoons olive oil, plus more for greasing the slow cooker
- 2½ pounds (1.1 kg) boneless lamb shoulder, cubed
- 4 tablespoons curry paste
- 5 garlic cloves, finely chopped
- 2 onions, roughly chopped
- Salt and freshly ground black pepper, to taste
- 1 lamb stock cube
- 2 tomatoes, chopped
- 2½ cups unsweetened coconut milk
- 1 cup water
- Fresh coriander, roughly chopped, for garnish
- Full-fat Greek yogurt, to serve

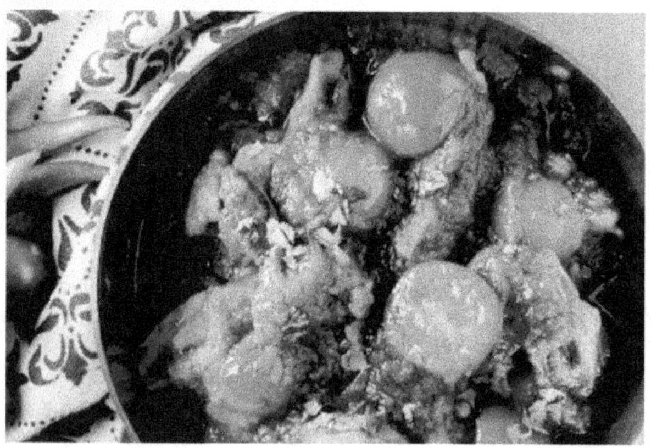

DIRECTIONS

1. Warm the olive oil in a nonstick skillet over medium-high heat.
2. Add and sear the lamb shoulder for 3 minutes until browned on both sides.
3. Grease the slow cooker with olive oil.
4. Place the cooked lamb into the slow cooker, and add the curry paste, garlic, onions, salt, and black pepper. Toss to coat the lamb well.
5. Add the stock cube, tomatoes, coconut milk, and water to the slow cooker. Stir to mix well.
6. Put the slow cooker lid on and cook on LOW for 8 hours.
7. Transfer the lamb curry to a large plate, and spread the coriander and yogurt on top to serve.

NUTRITIONS

- Calories: 406 kcal
- Total Fat: 28.2g
- Total Carbs: 10.5g
- Fiber: 4.3g
- Net Carbs: 6.2g
- Protein: 31.6g

20. GARLICKY LAMB LEG WITH ROSEMARY

PREPARATION TIME	COOK TIME	SERVING
15'	30'	8

INGREDIENTS

- 3 tablespoons extra-virgin olive oil
- 4 pounds (1.8 kg) boneless leg of lamb
- Salt and freshly ground black pepper, to taste
- 2 tablespoons chopped rosemary
- 1 tablespoon garlic
- 2 cups water

DIRECTIONS

1. Warm the olive oil in a nonstick skillet over medium-high heat.
2. Add the lamb leg to the skillet, and sprinkle with salt and black pepper. Sear for 3 minutes until browned on both sides.
3. Remove the lamb leg from the skillet to a platter. Allow it to cool for a few minutes, and then rub with the rosemary and garlic.
4. Pour the water into a pressure cooker with a steamer, and then arrange the lamb leg on the steamer.
5. Put the pressure cooker lid on and cook for 30 minutes.
6. Release the pressure, and remove the lamb leg from the pressure cooker. Allow cooling for 10 minutes and slice to serve.

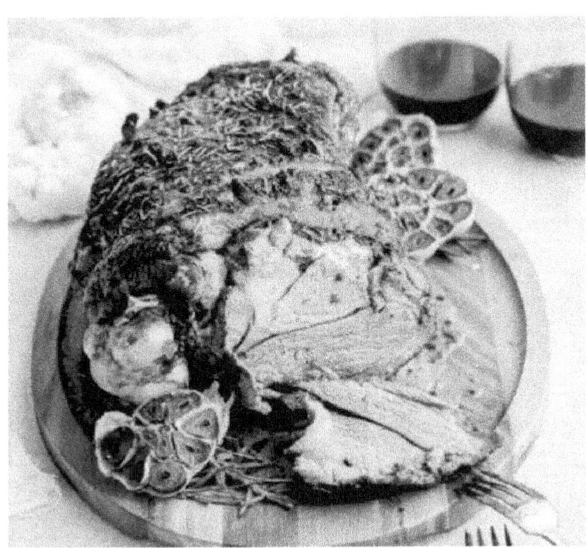

NUTRITIONS

- Calories: 366 kcal
- Total Fat: 16.2g
- Total Carbs: 1.2g
- Fiber: 0.6g
- Net Carbs: 0.6g
- Protein: 51.1g

9. APPETIZERS AND SNACKS

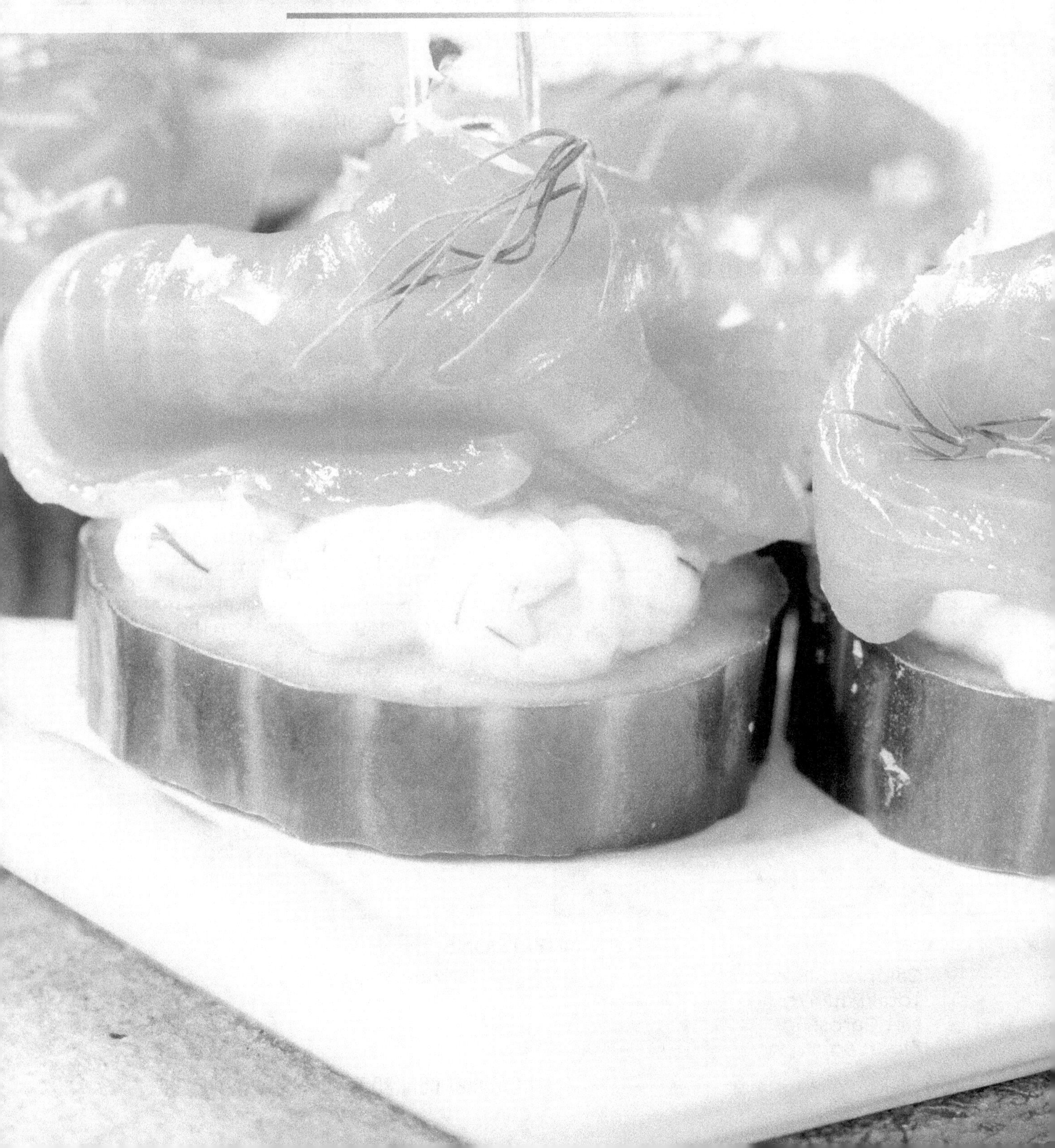

1. CARAMELIZED BUTTER WITH CREAMY EGGS

PREPARATION TIME
10'

COOK TIME
15'

SERVING
4T

INGREDIENTS

- 1.5 pounds (680 g) green asparagus
- 2 ounces (57 g) butter, melted
- 4 eggs
- ½ cup sour cream
- 3 ounces (85 g) parmesan cheese, grated
- Salt and cayenne pepper, to taste
- 1 tablespoon olive oil
- 3 ounces (85 g) butter
- 1½ tablespoons lemon juice

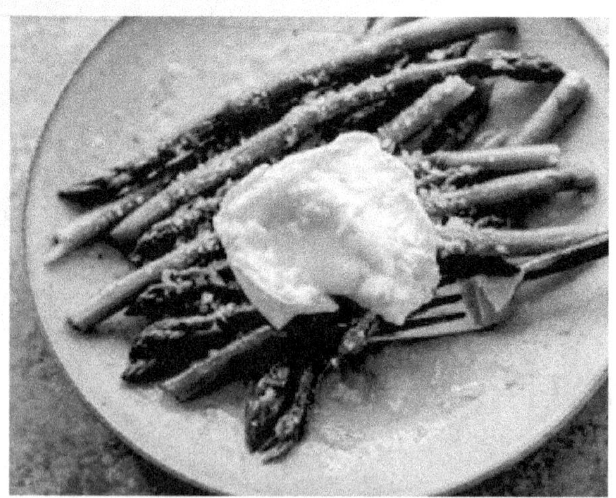

DIRECTIONS

1. Put the 2 ounces of melted butter in a nonstick skillet, and tilt the pan so the butter covers the bottom evenly. Add the eggs into the skillet and stir-fry over medium heat for 3 minutes or until the eggs are scrambled.
2. Transfer the scrambled eggs into a blender, and then add the sour cream and cheese. Process until the mixture is creamy, and then sprinkle the salt and cayenne pepper to season.
3. Clean the skillet and drizzle with olive oil then add the asparagus, salt, and cayenne pepper and roast over medium heat for 2 or 3 minutes or until it's soft. Flip the asparagus constantly during the cooking. Remove from the skillet and set aside.
4. Clean the skillet and put in 3 ounces of butter, then sauté for 8 minutes or until the butter is browned and smells nutty.
5. Add the lemon juice and cooked asparagus into the skillet and sauté with the browned butter for 2 to 3 minutes until warmed through.
6. Transfer to a serving plate, and top with creamy eggs before serving.

NUTRITIONS

- Calories: 518 kcal
- Total Fat: 47g
- Net Carbs: 6g
- Fiber: 4g
- Protein: 18 g

2. SIMPLE FLUFFY PANCAKES

 **PREPARATION TIME**
5'

 **COOK TIME**
15'

 **SERVING**
8

INGREDIENTS

- 1 egg
- 1¼ cups coconut milk
- 3 tablespoons butter, melted
- ½ cup coconut flour
- 3½ teaspoons baking powder
- ¼ tablespoon stevia
- 1 teaspoon salt

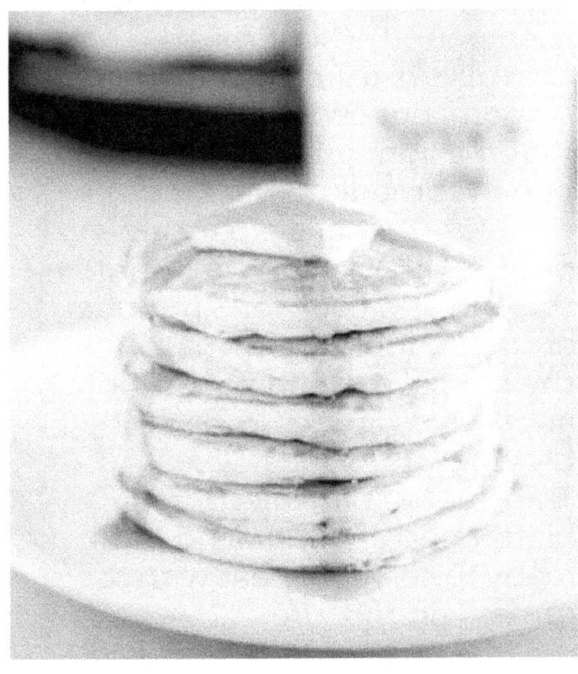

DIRECTIONS

1. Whisk together the egg, coconut milk, and butter in a large bowl. Combine the flour, baking powder, stevia, and salt in a separate bowl.
2. Pour the flour mixture into the egg mixture. Keep whisking until lumps are gone.
3. Warm a lightly greased baking pan over medium heat for 10 minutes. Make a pancake: Pour ¼ cup of the mixture in the pan and cook for 3 minutes or until bubbly. Flip the pancake over and cook for another 3 minutes until fluffy.
4. Transfer the pancake onto a platter and allow cooling until ready to serve. Repeat with the remaining mixture.

NUTRITIONS

- Calories: 171 kcal
- Total Fat: 14.6g
- Carbs: 9.5g
- Protein: 2.8g

- Cholesterol: 89mg
- Sodium: 346mg

3. SWEET AND SOUR PANCAKES

PREPARATION TIME	COOK TIME	SERVING
10'	20'	4

INGREDIENTS

- ¾ cup coconut milk
- 2 tablespoons white vinegar
- 1 egg, beaten
- 2 tablespoons butter, melted
- ¼ cup coconut flour or almond flour
- ½ teaspoon baking soda
- 1 teaspoon baking powder
- ¼ teaspoon liquid stevia
- ½ teaspoon salt

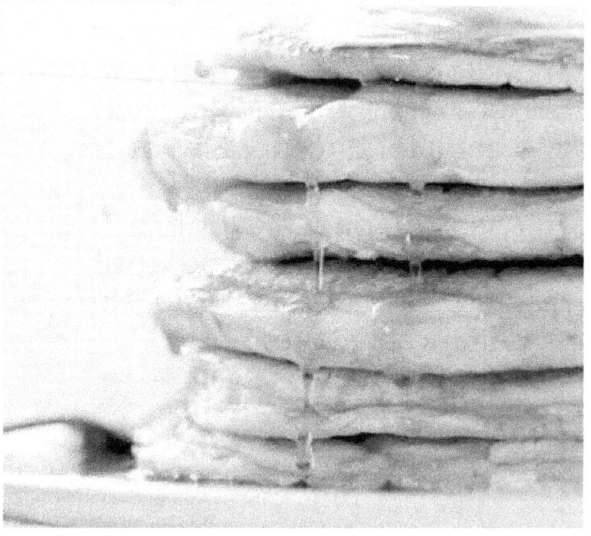

DIRECTIONS

1. Mix the milk with white vinegar in a bowl. Let it sit for 5 minutes till turning 'sour', then pour the beaten egg and melted butter into the bowl. Stir to mix well.
2. In a separate bowl, mix the coconut flour, baking soda, baking powder, stevia, and salt, then pour the flour mixture into the milk mixture. Fully stir until smooth, but avoid over-mixing.
3. Warm a lightly greased baking pan over medium heat for 10 minutes. To make a pancake, pour ¼ cup of the mixture into the pan and cook for 3 minutes or until bubbles form on top. Flip the pancake over and cook for another 3 minutes until lightly browned.
4. Transfer the pancake onto a platter and allow cooling until ready to serve. Repeat with the remaining mixture.

NUTRITIONS

- Calories: 216 kcal
- Total Fat: 19.0g
- Carbs: 8.7g
- Protein: 4.2g

- Cholesterol: 170mg
- Sodium: 526mg

4. BACON-WRAPPED JALAPENO

 **PREPARATION TIME**
10'

 **COOK TIME**
10'

 **SERVING**
6

INGREDIENTS

- 12 slices bacon
- 6 fresh jalapeño peppers, halved lengthwise and deseeded
- 1 (8 ounces/227 g) package cream cheese

DIRECTIONS

1. On a clean working surface, scatter the cream cheese on top of the jalapeño pepper halves.
2. Wrap each pepper half with a slice of bacon, and use a toothpick to secure. Repeat with the remaining pepper halves and bacon slices.
3. Arrange the bacon-wrapped jalapeño on a preheated grill and grill for 8 minutes, flipping the bacon halfway through or until lightly browned.
4. Remove from the grill, and discard the toothpick. Allow it to cool before serving.

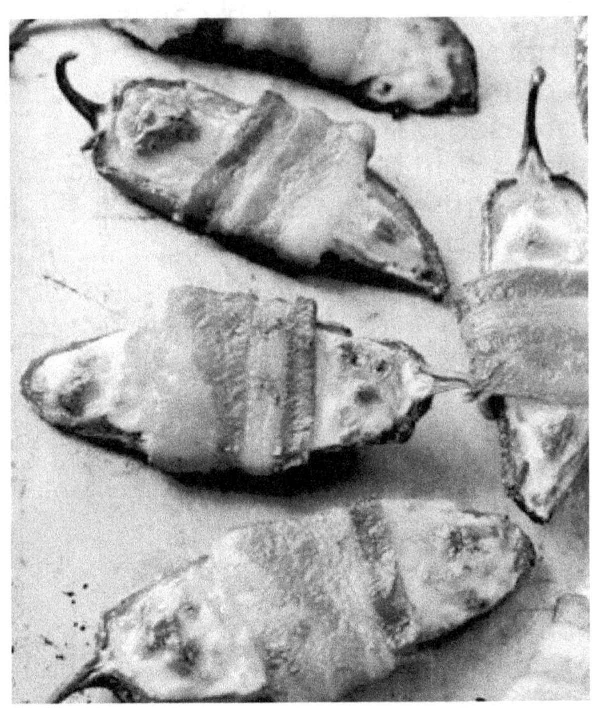

NUTRITIONS

- Calories: 391 kcal
- Total Fat: 38.3g kcal
- Carbs: 2.2g
- Protein: 9.5g

- Cholesterol: 79mg
- Sodium: 577mg

5. CHEESY SPINACH BROWNIES

 **PREPARATION TIME** 20'

 **COOK TIME** 35'

 **SERVING** 24

INGREDIENTS

- 1 (10-ounce/284 g) package spinach, blanched and chopped
- 1 cup almond flour
- 1 teaspoon gluten-free baking powder
- 1 teaspoon salt
- 2 eggs, beaten
- 1 cup unsweetened almond milk
- ½ cup butter, melted
- 1 (8 ounces/227 g) package mozzarella cheese, shredded
- 1 onion, chopped

DIRECTIONS

1. Start by preheating the oven to 375°F (190°C).
2. Make the brownies: Combine the flour, baking powder, and salt in a bowl. Add in the beaten eggs, almond milk, and melted butter. Then add the spinach, cheese, and onion. Stir to combine.
3. Pour the mixture into a lightly greased baking pan. Arrange the pan in the oven and bake for 30 minutes or until a toothpick inserted in the center of the brownies comes out clean.
4. Remove from the oven. Allow cooling for a few minutes and slice to serve.

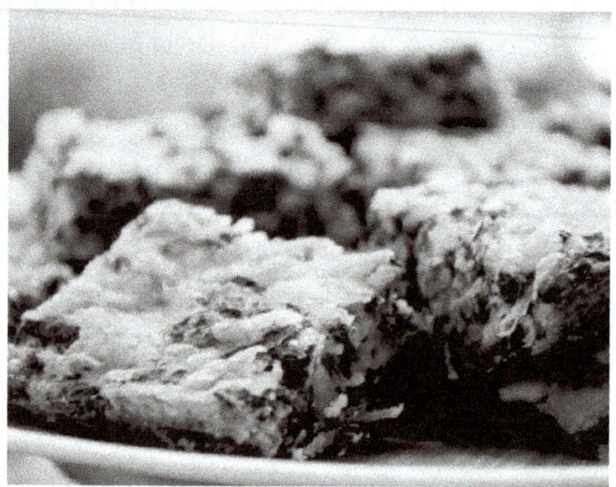

NUTRITIONS

- Calories: 92 kcal
- Total Fat: 6g
- Carbs: 5.6g
- Protein: 4.1g
- Cholesterol: 32mg
- Sodium: 216mg

6. CLOUD BREAD AND BLT

PREPARATION TIME	COOK TIME	SERVING
25'	20'	2

INGREDIENTS

Cloud bread:
- 3 eggs
- 1 pinch salt
- ¼ teaspoon cream of tartar (optional)
- ½ tablespoon ground psyllium husk powder
- 4 ounces (113 g) cream cheese
- ½ teaspoon gluten-free baking powder

Filling:
- 1 tomato, thinly sliced
- 2 ounces (57 g) lettuce, chopped
- 4 tablespoons sugar-free mayonnaise
- 5 ounces (142 g) bacon, cooked and diced

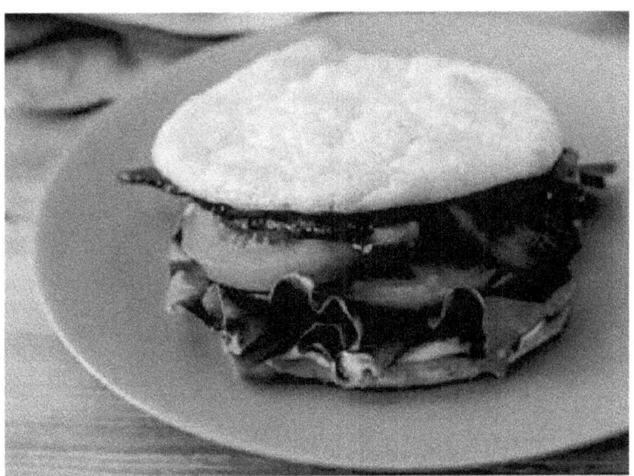

DIRECTIONS

1. Start by preheating the oven to 300°F (150°C).
2. Separate the eggs into a bowl of egg whites and another bowl of egg yolks. Sprinkle the egg whites with salt and cream of tartar, whip until puffed.
3. Then add the psyllium husk powder, cream cheese, and baking powder to the whipped egg whites. Pour the egg white mixture into the egg yolks, stir to mix well.
4. Line a baking pan with parchment paper, spoon two dollops on the mixture on the paper. Use a spatula to form dollops of the mixture into ½-inch (1.3 cm) thick.
5. Arrange the pan in the preheated oven and bake for 25 minutes, flipping the cloud bread halfway through the cooking time or until golden brown. Repeat with the remaining mixture and make two more cloud breads.
6. Assemble two pieces of the cloud breads with the ingredients for the filling according to your favorite order before serving.

NUTRITIONS

- Calories: 800 kcal
- Total Fat: 75g
- Net Carbs: 7g
- Fiber: 3g
- Protein: 22 g

7. FRIED BACON AND EGGS

PREPARATION TIME
10'

COOK TIME
10'

SERVING
4

INGREDIENTS

- 4 ounces (113 g) bacon, in slices
- 4 eggs
- Salt and ground black pepper, to taste

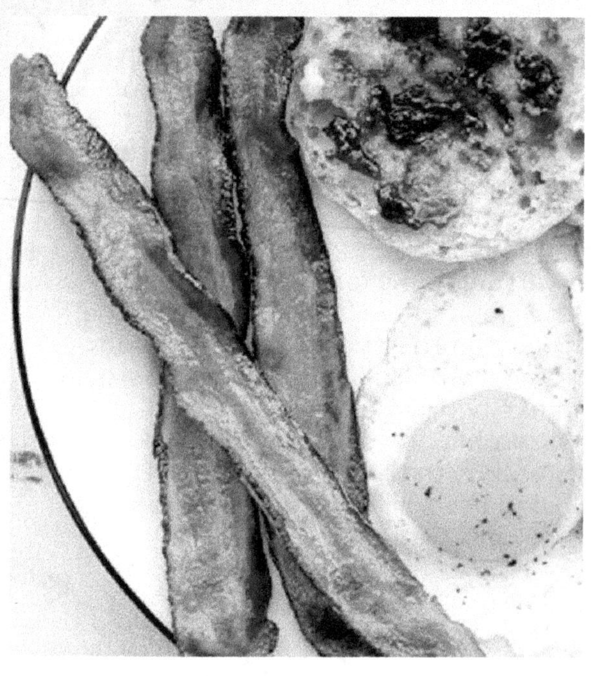

DIRECTIONS

1. Cook the bacon in a nonstick skillet over medium-high heat for 3 to 4 minutes. When it starts to buckle and curl, loosen and flip the bacon slice so that it browns evenly and cook for another 3 to 4 minutes.
2. Transfer the cooked bacon into a plate lined with paper towels. Leave the fat rendered from the bacon in the pan.
3. Break the eggs into the pan and fry over medium heat until they reach your desired doneness. Flip the eggs halfway through. You may need to work in batches to avoid overcrowding.
4. Add the bacon to the pan and cook with eggs, then sprinkle with salt and ground black pepper to taste, and cook for an additional minute.
5. Serve them warm on a platter.

NUTRITIONS

- Calories: 272 kcal
- Total Fat: 22g
- Net Carbs: 1g
- Fiber: 0g
- Protein: 15g

8. GUACAMOLE

PREPARATION TIME
10'

COOK TIME
0

SERVING
4

INGREDIENTS

- 3 avocados, peeled, pitted, and mashed
- 1 lime, juiced
- 1 teaspoon salt
- 2 tablespoons (plum) tomatoes, diced
- 3 tablespoons fresh cilantro, chopped
- ½ cup onion, diced
- 1 teaspoon garlic, minced
- 1 pinch ground cayenne pepper (optional)

DIRECTIONS

1. Combine the mashed avocados, lime juice, and salt in a large bowl, and then add in the tomato dices, chopped cilantro, diced onion, minced garlic, and cayenne pepper. Stir to combine well.
2. Wrap the bowl in plastic and store in the fridge for at least 1 hour before serving.

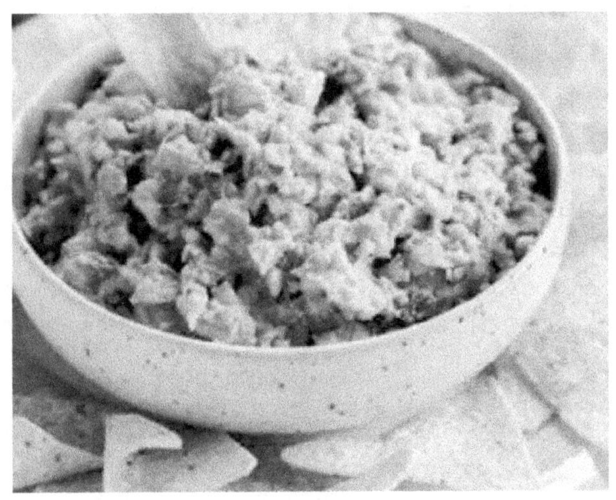

NUTRITIONS

- Calories: 262 kcal
- Total Fat: 22.3g
- Carbs: 18g
- Protein: 3.8g
- Cholesterol: 0mg
- Sodium: 596mg

9. HALLOUMI CHEESE WITH SCRAMBLED EGGS

PREPARATION TIME
10'

COOK TIME
15

SERVING
2

INGREDIENTS

- 3 ounces (85 g) halloumi cheese, diced
- 4 ounces (113 g) bacon, diced
- 4 eggs
- 4 tablespoons fresh parsley, chopped
- Salt and ground black pepper, to taste
- 2 scallions, chopped
- 2 ounces (57 g) olives, pitted

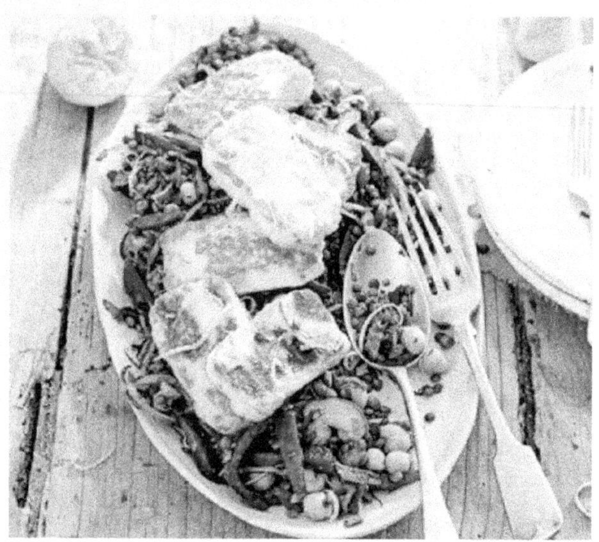

DIRECTIONS

1. Whisk together the eggs, parsley, salt, and ground black pepper in a medium bowl. Set aside.
2. Cook the bacon in a nonstick skillet over medium-high heat for 3 to 4 minutes. When it starts to buckle and curl, loosen and flip the bacon slice so that it browns evenly and cook for another 3 to 4 minutes.
3. Use the spatula to dice the bacon, then add the halloumi cheese and scallions, cook for 1 more minute.
4. Add the egg mixture and olives into the skillet, then turn down the heat and sauté over medium heat for 3 minutes until the eggs are scrambled.
5. Serve them on a platter immediately.

NUTRITIONS

- Calories: 657 kcal
- Total Fat: 59g
- Net Carbs: 4g
- Fiber: 1g
- Protein: 28 g

10. JALAPEÑO PEPPERS STUFFED WITH SAUSAGE

PREPARATION TIME
10'

COOK TIME
7'

SERVING
12

INGREDIENTS

- 1 pound (454 g) large fresh jalapeño peppers, halved lengthwise and deseeded
- 1 pound (454 g) ground pork sausage
- 1 cup Parmesan cheese, shredded
- 1 (8 ounces/227 g) package cream cheese, softened
- 1 (8 ounces/227 g) bottle Ranch dressing (optional)

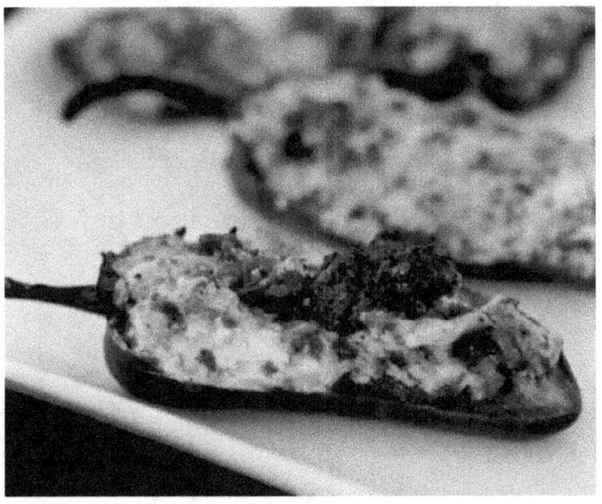

DIRECTIONS

1. Start by preheating the oven to 425°F (220°C).
2. Sauté the ground pork sausage in a nonstick skillet over medium-high heat for 6 minutes or until lightly browned. Transfer to a plate lined with paper towels.
3. Combine the sautéed sausage with parmesan cheese and cream cheese. Scoop 1 tablespoon of this mixture into each jalapeño half, and then place them into a greased baking pan. You may need to work in batches to avoid overcrowding. Transfer the pan into the preheated oven.
4. Bake for 20 minutes or until the jalapeño peppers are blistered and the sausage mixture is well browned, then top them with Ranch dressing, if desired, and bake for 2 more minutes.
5. Remove from the oven. Allow cooling for a few minutes before serving.

NUTRITIONS

- Calories: 362 kcal
- Total Fat: 34.3g
- Carbs: 4.3g
- Protein: 9.2g

- Cholesterol: 58mg
- Sodium: 601mg

11. KETO SPINACH AND BACON FRITTATA

PREPARATION TIME
10'

COOK TIME
35'

SERVING
4T

INGREDIENTS

- 8 ounces (227 g) fresh spinach, chopped
- 5 ounces (142 g) bacon
- 2 tablespoons butter
- 8 eggs, beaten
- 1 cup heavy whipping cream
- 5 ounces (142 g) mozzarella cheese, shredded
- Salt and ground black pepper, to taste

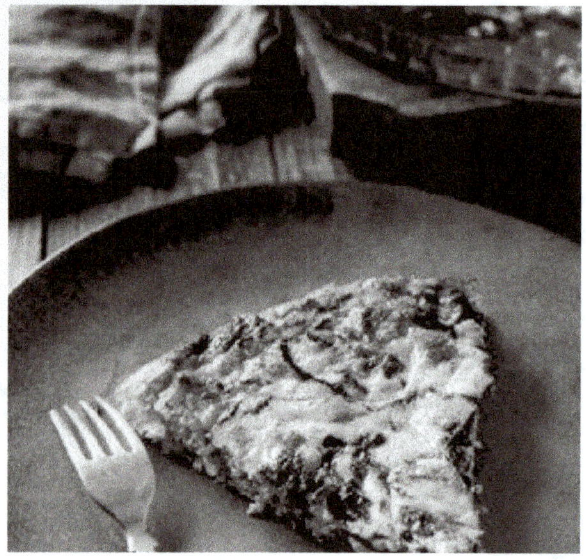

DIRECTIONS

1. Start by preheating the oven to 350°F (180°C).
2. Cook the bacon in a nonstick skillet over medium-high heat for 3 to 4 minutes. When it starts to buckle and curl, loosen and flip the bacon slice so that it browns evenly and cook for another 3 to 4 minutes.
3. Use a spatula to dice the bacon, then add the butter into the skillet and melt. Tilt the skillet so the butter coats the bottom evenly.
4. Add the spinach into the skillet and sauté until wilted, then transfer them into a greased baking pan.
5. To make the frittata, combine the beaten eggs and cream in a bowl, then pour the mixture into the pan. Arrange the pan in the preheated oven.
6. Bake the frittata for 25 minutes. You can check the doneness by cutting a small slit in the center, if raw eggs run into the cut continue baking for another few minutes.
7. Sprinkle with mozzarella cheese, salt, and ground black pepper, and bake for another 2 minutes until the cheese melts.
8. Remove the frittata from the oven, allow to cool for a few minutes before serving.

NUTRITIONS

- Calories: 661 kcal
- Total Fat: 59g
- Net Carbs: 4g
- Fiber: 1g
- Protein: 27g

12. MUSHROOM AND YELLOW ONION OMELET

 **PREPARATION TIME**
5'

 **COOK TIME**
10'

 **SERVING**
1

INGREDIENTS

- 4 large mushrooms, sliced
- ¼ cup yellow onion, chopped
- 3 eggs
- Salt and ground black pepper, to taste
- 1 ounce (28 g) butter, melted
- 1 ounce (28 g) cheddar cheese, shredded

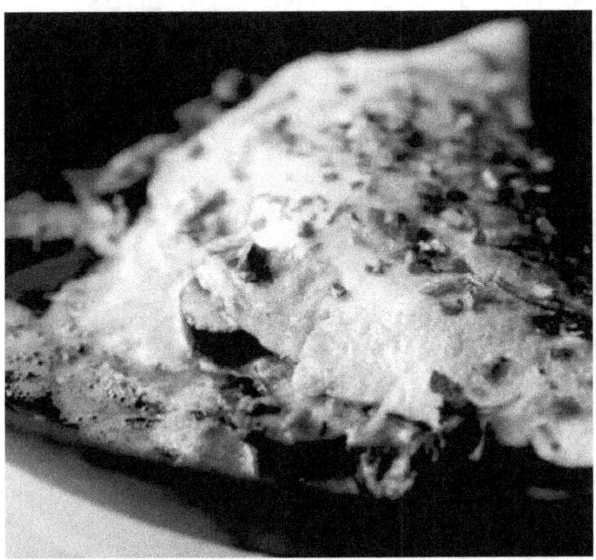

DIRECTIONS

1. Whisk the eggs in a large bowl, and sprinkle with salt and ground black pepper. Stir until it's frothy. Set aside.
2. Drizzle the melted butter in a nonstick skillet. Tilt the pan so the butter covers the bottom evenly. Sauté the mushrooms and yellow onion in the skillet over medium-high heat for 3 minutes until the mushrooms are tender and the onion is translucent.
3. To make the omelet, pour the egg mixture over the skillet and cook for 1 to 2 minutes until the omelet starts to firm, then flip the omelet, sprinkle with cheddar cheese, and cook for another 1 minute.
4. Gently fold the omelet in half with a spatula and transfer to a plate to cool before serving.

NUTRITIONS

- Calories: 517 kcal
- Total Fat: 44g
- Net Carbs: 5g
- Fiber: 1g
- Protein: 26 g

13. PARMESAN-CRUSTED ASPARAGUS

 **PREPARATION TIME**
10'

 **COOK TIME**
15'

 **SERVING**
4

INGREDIENTS

- 1 ounce (28 g) shaved parmesan cheese
- 1 pound (454 g) thin asparagus spears
- 1 tablespoon extra-virgin olive oil
- Freshly ground black pepper, to taste

DIRECTIONS

1. Start by preheating the oven to 450°F (220°C).
2. Coat a baking pan with olive oil, then place the asparagus spears into the pan. Sprinkle it with parmesan cheese and ground black pepper.
3. Arrange the pan in the preheated oven and cook for 12 minutes until the asparagus spears are crisp and tender, and the cheese melts.
4. Remove them from the oven. Allow it to cool for a few minutes before serving.

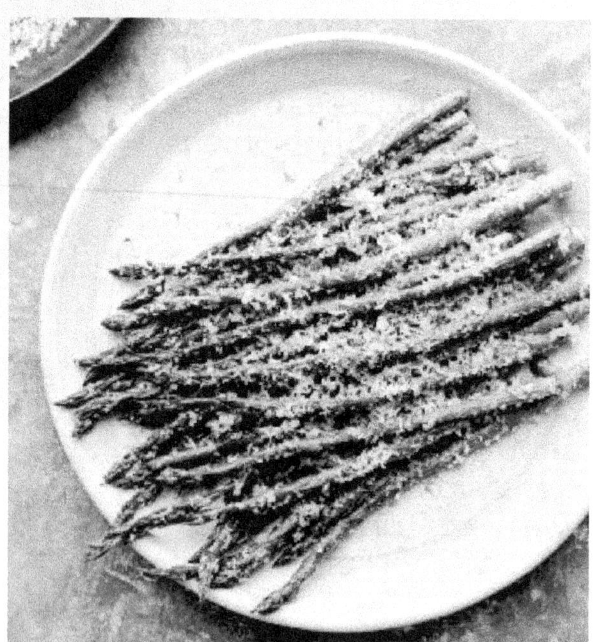

NUTRITIONS

- Calories: 93 kcal
- Total Fat: 5.6g
- Carbs: 7g
- Protein: 5.3g

- Cholesterol: 6mg
- Sodium: 114mg
- T

14. LOW-CARB CHEESY OMELET

PREPARATION TIME
5'

COOK TIME
10'

SERVING
2

INGREDIENTS

- 6 eggs
- 7 ounces (198 g) shredded Cheddar cheese
- Salt and ground black pepper, to taste
- 3 ounces (85 g) butter

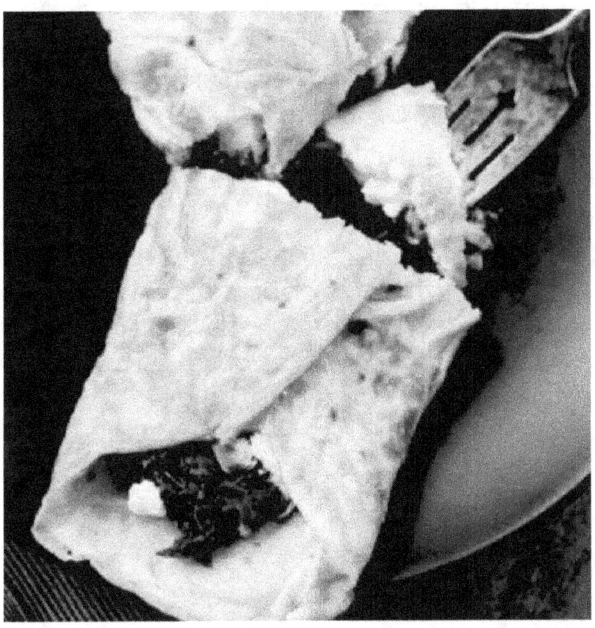

DIRECTIONS

1. In a bowl, whisk all the eggs until they are frothy and smooth. Add half of the cheddar cheese and blend well.
2. Add the pepper and salt to season.
3. In a frying pan, melt the butter over medium-high heat, then pour the egg mixture and cook for a few minutes until you see the eggs at the edges of the pan beginning to set.
4. Reduce the heat to low as you continue cooking the mixture for 3 minutes until it is almost cooked. Flip the omelet halfway through the cooking time. Scatter the remaining cheese on top and cook for another 1 to 2 minutes until the cheese melts.
5. Fold your omelet and serve while warm.

NUTRITIONS

- Calories: 899 kcal
- Total Fat: 79g
- Fiber: 0g
- Net Carbs: 5g
- Protein: 39.2g

15. SWEET CREAMY CAULIFLOWER

 **PREPARATION TIME** 15'

 **COOK TIME** 30'

 **SERVING** 6

INGREDIENTS

- 1 large head cauliflower, cut into bite-sized pieces
- 1 cup shredded mozzarella cheese
- ½ cup keto-friendly mayonnaise
- ½ cup sour cream
- 3 tablespoons chopped fresh chives
- ¼ cup bacon bits
- 1 cup shredded sharp Cheddar cheese

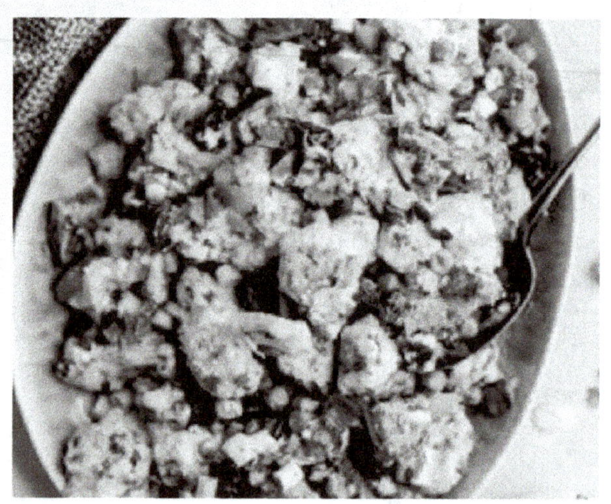

DIRECTIONS

1. Start by preheating the oven to 425°F (220°C).
2. Put a steamer insert into your saucepan then fill the saucepan with water up to a level slightly above the bottom of the steamer. Boil the water.
3. Add the cauliflower to the steamer. Cover the lid and steam for 10 minutes or until tender. Drain and cool for 10 minutes
4. In a large bowl, mix the mozzarella cheese, mayonnaise, sour cream, chives, and half of the bacon bits. Add the cauliflower and stir to combine well.
5. Pour the mixture into a baking dish. Sprinkle with the cheddar cheese and the remaining bits of bacon.
6. Place it in the oven and bake for about 20 minutes or until golden brown and all the cheese melts.
7. Transfer to six serving plates. Allow cooling for a few minutes before serving.

NUTRITIONS

- Calories: 366 kcal
- Total Fat: 30.1g
- Carbs: 9.5g
- Protein: 15.7g
- Cholesterol: 53mg
- Sodium: 564mg

16. FAUX POTATO (CAULIFLOWER) SALAD

PREPARATION TIME
25'

COOK TIME
10'

SERVING
8T

INGREDIENTS

- 16 cups (2080 g) water
- 2 tablespoons salt
- 1 (30 ounces/850 g) head cauliflower, cut into bite-sized pieces
- 1 cup mayonnaise, keto-friendly
- ½ cup thinly sliced celery
- 3 slices cooked bacon, crumbled
- 4 tablespoons minced onion
- 3 tablespoons unsweetened pickles, minced
- 1 teaspoon spicy mustard, or to taste
- ⅛ teaspoon ground turmeric
- 2 hard-boiled eggs, diced
- Salt and ground black pepper, to taste

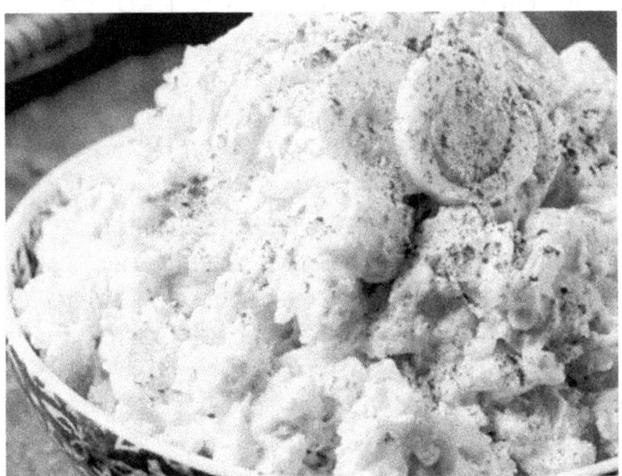

DIRECTIONS

1. Prepare a pot of salted water. Bring it to a boil and add the cauliflower. Cook for 3 minutes or until the cauliflower is fork-tender. Drain the vegetable through a colander and set aside to cool.
2. Spread the cauliflower on a large platter and refrigerate for about 20 minutes.
3. Meanwhile, mix the remaining ingredients except for the eggs, salt, and black pepper in a large bowl. After 20 minutes, stir in the cauliflower and eggs. Season with salt and black pepper, and then serve.

NUTRITIONS

- Calories: 348 kcal
- Total Fat: 29.7g
- Carbs: 10.6g
- Protein: 10.6g
- Cholesterol: 63mg
- Sodium: 2001mg

17. CHICKEN TONNATO SALAD

PREPARATION TIME
10'

COOK TIME
20'

SERVING
4

INGREDIENTS

Tonnato sauce:
- 4 ounces (113 g) tuna in olive oil
- 2 garlic cloves, minced
- ¼ cup chopped fresh basil
- 1 teaspoon dried parsley
- 2 tablespoons lemon juice
- ½ cup mayonnaise, keto-friendly
- ¼ cup olive oil
- ½ teaspoon salt
- ¼ teaspoon black pepper

Chicken:
- 1.5 pounds (680 g) chicken breasts
- 4 cups water
- 1 teaspoon salt
- 7 ounces (198 g) leafy greens

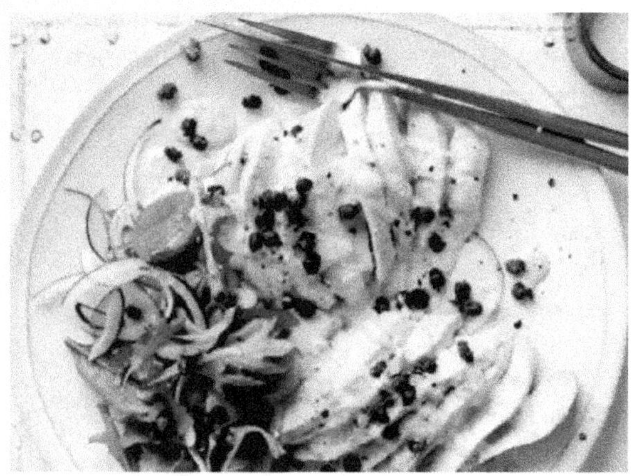

DIRECTIONS

1. Make the tonnato sauce: Add all the sauce's ingredients to a bowl and use an immersion blender to process until smooth. Set the dressing aside and let the flavors combine.
2. Make the salad: Place the chicken in a pot and cover with slightly salted water. If using pre-cooked chicken for the salad, this step won't be needed.
3. Boil the chicken over medium heat while scooping off and discarding the foam that floats on top. Reduce the heat and simmer for 15 minutes or until the chicken is cooked through or it reaches an internal temperature of 165°F (74°C).
4. Use tongs to remove the chicken breasts onto a flat surface. Let them cool for 10 minutes before slicing.
5. Spread the leafy greens on a serving platter, top with the chicken, and drizzle the dressing all over the salad.

NUTRITIONS

- Calories: 678 kcal
- Total Fat: 53.2g
- Net Carbs: 2g
- Fiber: 2g
- Protein: 45.2g

18. DILL DRESSED TOMATO AND CUCUMBER SALAD

PREPARATION TIME	COOK TIME	SERVING
15'	0	6T

INGREDIENTS

- ¼ cup apple cider vinegar
- 1½ teaspoon erythritol
- ½ teaspoon salt
- ½ teaspoon chopped fresh dill weed
- ¼ teaspoon ground black pepper
- 2 tablespoons olive oil
- 2 (4 ounces/113 g) cucumbers, sliced
- 1 cup sliced red onion
- 2 ripe tomatoes, cut into wedges

DIRECTIONS

1. In a large bowl, whisk the vinegar, erythritol, salt, dill weed, black pepper, and olive oil.
2. Add the cucumbers, red onion, tomatoes, and toss adequately. Serve.

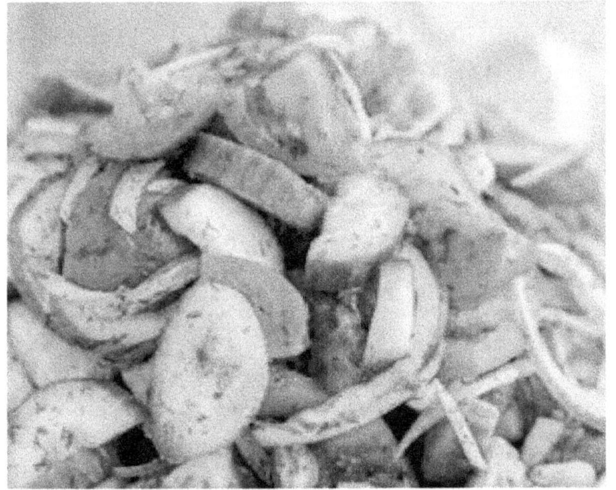

NUTRITIONS

- Calories: 70 kcal
- Total Fat: 4.7g
- Carbs: 7.2g
- Protein: 1g
- Cholesterol: 0mg
- Sodium: 199mg

19. CREAMY BROCCOLI SALAD

PREPARATION TIME
25'

COOK TIME
10'

SERVING
4

INGREDIENTS

- 1 pound (454 g) bacon, chopped
- 2 cups broccoli, cut into florets
- 2 cups cauliflower, cut into florets
- ¼ cup chopped green onions
- ½ cup mayonnaise, keto-friendly
- ¼ cup distilled white vinegar
- 1 tablespoon sour cream
- 1 pinch garlic powder
- 1 pinch dried basil
- ¼ cup shredded Cheddar cheese
- 1 tablespoon chopped fresh cilantro, or to taste

DIRECTIONS

1. Cook bacon in a nonstick skillet over medium heat for 5 minutes or until crispy and golden brown. Transfer to a plate and set aside.
2. In a large bowl, mix the broccoli, cauliflower, and green onions.
3. In a small bowl, whisk the mayonnaise, vinegar, sour cream, garlic powder, and basil. Mix the dressing with the broccoli salad until well coated. Place the salad in the fridge to chill for 1 hour to let the flavors blend in.
4. Garnish with the cheddar cheese and cilantro. Serve immediately.

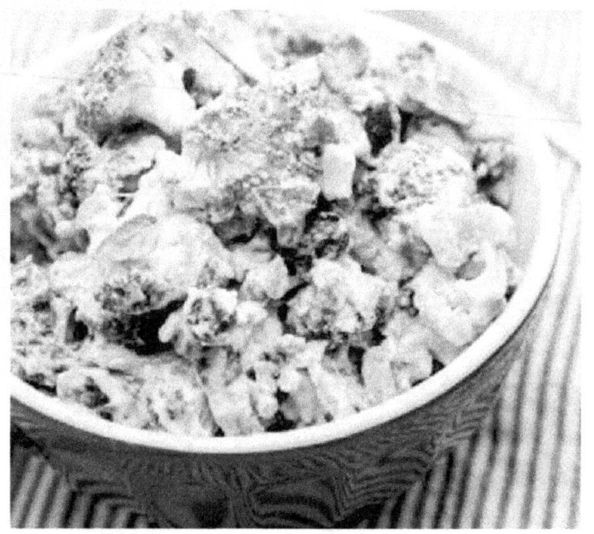

NUTRITIONS

- Calories: 531 kcal
- Total Fat: 45.9g
- Carbs: 12g
- Protein: 17.4g
- Cholesterol: 60mg
- Sodium: 1106mg

KETO DIET COOKBOOK FOR WOMEN OVER 50

20. SHRIMP SKEWERS

PREPARATION TIME	COOK TIME	SERVING
70'	0	6

INGREDIENTS

- 2 pounds (907 g) fresh shrimp, peeled and deveined
- 2 tablespoons red wine vinegar
- ¼ cup unsweetened tomato sauce
- 3 garlic cloves, minced
- ⅓ cup olive oil
- 2 tablespoons fresh basil, chopped
- ½ teaspoon salt
- ¼ teaspoon cayenne pepper

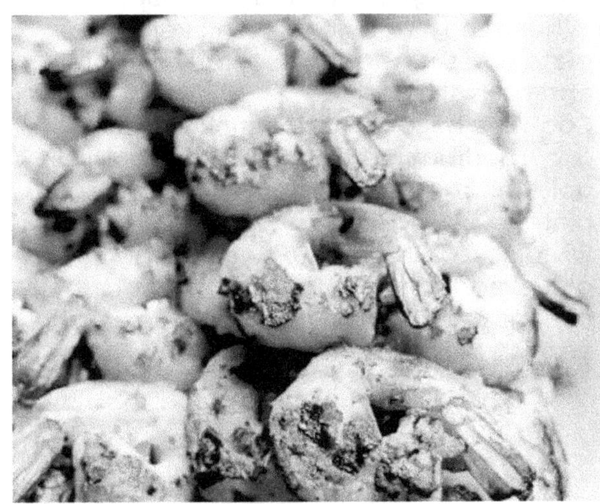

DIRECTIONS

1. Combine the red wine vinegar, tomato sauce, garlic, and olive oil in a large bowl. Put the peeled and deveined shrimps in the bowl, and sprinkle with basil, salt, and cayenne pepper. Toss to coat well.
2. Wrap the bowl in plastic and refrigerate to marinate for at least 1 hour.
3. Discard the marinade. Thread the shrimps through the skewers, and then arrange the shrimp skewers onto a preheated grill.
4. Grill for 6 minutes. Flip halfway through the cooking time or until opaque. Serve warm.

NUTRITIONS

- Calories: 273 kcal
- Total Fat: 14.7g
- Carbs: 2.8g
- Protein: 31g
- Cholesterol: 230mg
- Sodium: 472mg

21. CHICKEN CAESAR SALAD

PREPARATION TIME
15'

COOK TIME
20'

SERVING
2

INGREDIENTS

DressinTg:
- ½ cup mayonnaise, keto-friendly
- 1 tablespoon Dijon mustard
- ½ lemon, zest and juice
- 0.5 ounce (14 g) parmesan cheese, finely grated
- 2 tablespoons finely chopped filets of anchovies
- 1 garlic clove, pressed or finely chopped
- Salt and black pepper to taste

Salad:
- 12 ounces (340 g) chicken breasts
- Salt and black pepper
- 1 tablespoon olive oil or melted butter
- 3 ounces (85 g) bacon, chopped
- 7 ounces (198 g) Romaine lettuce, chopped
- 1 ounce (28 g) Parmesan cheese, freshly grated

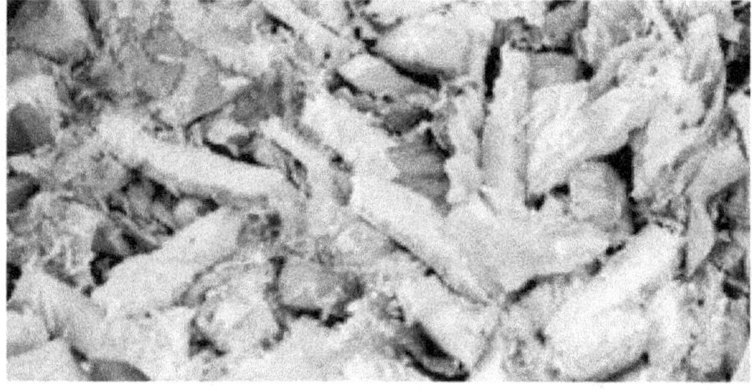

DIRECTIONS

1. Start by preheating the oven to 350°F (180°C).
2. Make the dressing: Add all the dressing's ingredients to a bowl and whisk until well combined. Place in the refrigerator for at least 15 minutes while you prepare the salad.
3. Make the salad: Season the chicken with salt, black pepper, and arrange on a baking sheet. Drizzle with olive oil or melted butter and bake in the oven for 20 minutes or until the chicken cooks through. (The chicken could also be cooked in a grill pan on a stovetop).
4. When ready, transfer the chicken to a plate and set aside to cool for 2 minutes, and then slice.
5. Cook the bacon in a nonstick skillet over medium heat for 5 minutes or until golden brown and crispy. Transfer to a plate.
6. Divide the lettuce onto two serving plates and top with the chicken and bacon. Drizzle with the dressing and garnish with parmesan cheese.

NUTRITIONS

- Calories: 1018 kcal
- Total Fat: 87.2g
- Net Carbs: 4.1g
- Fiber: 3g
- Protein: 51.2g

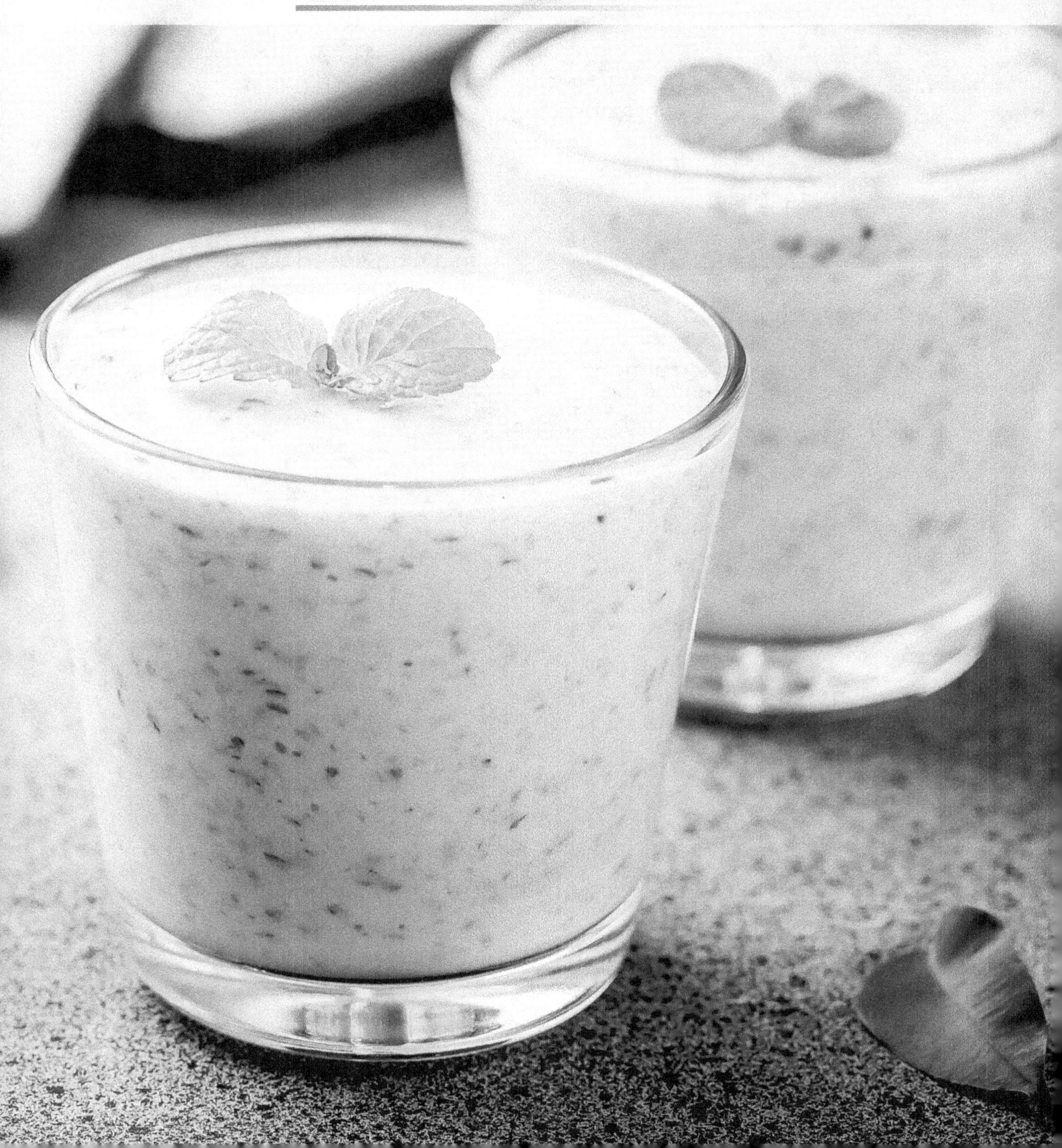

10. SNACKS AND SMOOTHIES RECIPES

1. VANILLA SMOOTHIE

PREPARATION TIME
5'

COOK TIME
0

SERVING
2T

INGREDIENTS

- 1 tablespoon organic vanilla extract
- 3–4 drops liquid stevia
- 1 cup heavy cream
- 1 ⅓ cups unsweetened almond milk
- ¼ cup ice cubes

DIRECTIONS

1. In a high-speed blender, put all the ingredients and blend until creamy.
2. Pour the smoothie into two glasses and serve immediately.

NUTRITIONS

- Calories: 252 kcal
- Net Carbs: 0g
- Total Fat: 24.5g
- Saturated Fat: 14g
- Cholesterol: 82mg
- Sodium: 143mg
- Total Carbs: 3.8g
- Fiber: 0.7g
- Sugar: 0.9g
- Protein: 1.9g

2. TURMERIC SMOOTHIE

PREPARATION TIME	COOK TIME	SERVING
10'	0	2

INGREDIENTS

- 2 ounces smoked salmon
- 1 lemon slice
- 4 olives
- 1 teaspoon pink peppercorns, crushed lightly
- 1 handful arugula salad leaves, fresh

DIRECTIONS

1. In a high-speed blender, put all the ingredients and blend until creamy.
2. Pour the smoothie into two glasses and serve immediately.

NUTRITIONS

- Calories: 179 kcal
- Net Carbs: 3.2g
- Total Fat: 19.9g
- Saturated Fat: 14.6g
- Cholesterol: 0mg
- Sodium: 159mg
- Total Carbs: 7.9g
- Fiber: 4.7g
- Sugar: 0.1g
- Protein: 2.7g

3. COFFEE SMOOTHIE

PREPARATION TIME	COOK TIME	SERVING
10'	0	2

INGREDIENTS

- 1 cup brewed coffee
- 2 tablespoons MCT oil
- 1 teaspoon vanilla extract
- ⅛ teaspoon stevia powder
- 1 cup heavy cream
- 1 cup ice cubes

DIRECTIONS

1. In a high-speed blender, put all the ingredients and blend until creamy.
2. Pour the smoothie into two glasses and serve immediately.

NUTRITIONS

- Calories: 314 kcal
- Net Carbs: 1.9g
- Total Fat: 36.2g
- Saturated Fat: 27.8g
- Cholesterol: 82mg
- Sodium: 29mg
- Total Carbs: 1.9g
- Fiber: 0g
- Sugar: 0.3g
- Protein: 1.4g

4. TMOCHA SMOOTHIE

PREPARATION TIME	COOK TIME	SERVING
10'	0	3

INGREDIENTS

- 1 large avocado; peeled, pitted, and chopped roughly
- 3 tablespoons cacao powder
- 2 teaspoons instant coffee crystals
- 3 tablespoons granulated erythritol
- 1 teaspoon organic vanilla extract
- ½ cup heavy cream
- 1½ cup unsweetened almond milk
- ½ cup ice cubes

DIRECTIONS

1. In a high-speed blender, put all the ingredients and blend until creamy.
2. Pour the smoothie into three glasses and serve immediately.

NUTRITIONS

- Calories: 208 kcal
- Net Carbs: 3.1g
- Total Fat: 19.9g
- Saturated Fat: 7.4g
- Cholesterol: 27mg
- Sodium: 101mg
- Total Carbs: 8.5g
- Fiber: 5.4g
- Sugar: 0.5g
- Protein: 2.9g

5. STRAWBERRY SMOOTHIE

PREPARATION TIME
10'

COOK TIME
0

SERVING
2

INGREDIENTS

- ½ cup fresh strawberries, hulled
- 8–10 fresh basil leaves
- 3–4 drops liquid stevia
- ½ cup plain Greek yogurt
- 1 cup unsweetened almond milk
- ¼ cup ice cubes

DIRECTIONS

1. In a high-speed blender, put all the ingredients and blend until creamy.
2. Pour the smoothie into two glasses and serve immediately.

NUTRITIONS

- Calories: 72 kcal
- Net Carbs: 4.8g
- Total Fat: 2.6g
- Saturated Fat: 0.7g
- Cholesterol: 5mg
- Sodium: 115mg
- Total Carbs: 6.1g
- Fiber: 1.3g
- Sugar: 3.5g
- Protein: 6.5g

6. RASPBERRY SMOOTHIE

PREPARATION TIME
10'

COOK TIME
0

SERVING
2

INGREDIENTS

- ¾ cup fresh blackberries
- 2 scoops unsweetened protein powder
- 1 teaspoon organic vanilla extract
- 1 teaspoon MCT oil
- 1¾ cups unsweetened almond milk
- ¼ cup ice cubes

DIRECTIONS

1. In a high-speed blender, put all the ingredients and blend until creamy.
2. Pour the smoothie into two glasses and serve immediately.

NUTRITIONS

- Calories: 215 kcal
- Net Carbs: 3.6g
- Total Fat: 9.1g
- Saturated Fat: 4.9g
- Cholesterol: 0mg
- Sodium: 422mg
- Total Carbs: 7.5g
- Fiber: 3.9g
- Sugar: 2.3g
- Protein: 26.8g

7. BLACKBERRY SMOOTHIE

PREPARATION TIME	COOK TIME	SERVING
10'	0	2

INGREDIENTS

- 2 ounces fresh blackberries
- 2 ounces cream cheese, softened
- 2 teaspoons erythritol
- ½ teaspoon organic vanilla extract
- ¼ cup heavy cream
- ¾ cup unsweetened almond milk
- ½ cup ice

DIRECTIONS

1. In a high-speed blender, put all the ingredients and blend until creamy.
2. Pour the smoothie into two glasses and serve immediately.

NUTRITIONS

- Calories: 181 kcal
- Net Carbs: 0g
- Total Fat: 16.9g
- Saturated Fat: 9.8g
- Cholesterol: 52mg
- Sodium: 159mg
- Total Carbs: 4.8g
- Fiber: 1.9g
- Sugar: 1.6g
- Protein: 3.2g

8. BLUEBERRY & SPINACH SMOOTHIE

PREPARATION TIME
10'

COOK TIME
0

SERVING
2

INGREDIENTS

- ¾ cup fresh spinach
- ½ cup frozen blueberries
- 1 tablespoon ground flaxseed
- ¼ cup full-fat Greek yogurt
- 1 cup unsweetened almond milk
- ¼ cup ice cubes

DIRECTIONS

1. In a high-speed blender, put all the ingredients and blend until creamy.
2. Pour the smoothie into two glasses and serve immediately.

NUTRITIONS

- Calories: 83 kcal
- Net Carbs: 6.2g
- Total Fat: 3.6g
- Saturated Fat: 0.7g
- Cholesterol: 1mg
- Sodium: 109mg
- Total Carbs: 8.8g
- Fiber: 2.6g
- Sugar: :4.8g
- Protein: 4.6g

9. GREEN SMOOTHIE

PREPARATION TIME
10'

COOK TIME
0

SERVING
2

INGREDIENTS

- 1 cup frozen avocado, peeled and pitted
- ¾ of English cucumber, peeled and chopped roughly
- 1 cup fresh baby spinach
- ½ cup fresh cilantro
- 1 (1-inch) piece fresh ginger, peeled
- ½ of lemon, peeled
- 1 cup cold water

DIRECTIONS

1. In a high-speed blender, put all the ingredients and blend until creamy.
2. Pour the smoothie into two glasses and serve immediately.

NUTRITIONS

- Calories: 164 kcal
- Net Carbs: 3g
- Total Fat: 14.5g
- Saturated Fat: 3g
- Cholesterol: 0mg
- Sodium: 23mg
- Total Carbs: 9g
- Fiber: 6g
- Sugar: 1.6g
- Protein: 2.4g

10. MATCHA SMOOTHIE

 **PREPARATION TIME**
5'

 **COOK TIME**
0

 **SERVING**
2

INGREDIENTS

- 2 tablespoons chia seeds
- 2 teaspoons matcha green tea powder
- ½ teaspoon fresh lemon juice
- 6–8 drops liquid stevia
- ¼ cup plain Greek yogurt
- 1½ cups unsweetened almond milk
- ¼ cup ice cubes

DIRECTIONS

1. In a high-speed blender, put all the ingredients and blend until creamy.
2. Pour the smoothie into two glasses and serve immediately.

NUTRITIONS

- Calories: 81 kcal
- Net Carbs: 0g
- Total Fat: 5.7g
- Saturated Fat: 0.9g
- Cholesterol: 1mg
- Sodium: 145mg
- Total Carbs: 5.7g
- Fiber: 3.3g
- Sugar: 1.2g
- Protein: 5.1g

PREPARATION TIME
15'

COOK TIME
25'

SERVING
4

INGREDIENTS

- 1 (10-ounce) bag fresh spinach leaves
- 1 tablespoon water
- 2 tablespoons olive oil
- 1 tablespoon garlic, minced
- 1 tablespoon fresh parsley, minced
- 4 ounces feta cheese, crumbled
- 4 ounces Monterey Jack cheese, shredded
- 1 (3-ounce) package cream cheese, softened
- Ground black pepper, to taste
- 2 tablespoons parmesan cheese, shredded

DIRECTIONS

1. Preheat your oven to 375°F.
2. In a large nonstick skillet, place spinach and water over high heat and cook for about 2–3 minutes, tossing with tongs.
3. Remove the spinach from heat and immediately place it in the bowl of ice water.
4. Drain the spinach and squeeze out the excess water.
5. Now, chop the spinach and set aside.
6. Heat oil in a small skillet over medium heat and sauté the garlic for about 1 minute.
7. Add parsley and sauté for about 15–20 seconds.
8. In the bowl of an electric mixer, add feta, Monterey Jack, cream cheese, and mix until well combined.
9. Add the spinach, garlic mixture, and black pepper, and mix to combine.
10. Place the spinach mixture into a baking dish evenly and sprinkle with Parmesan cheese.
11. Bake for approximately 20 minutes or until the top becomes golden.

NUTRITIONS

- Calories: 345 kcal
- Net Carbs: 0g
- Total Fat: 30g
- Saturated Fat: 15.8g
- Cholesterol: 76mg
- Sodium: 631mg
- Total Carbs: 5.4g
- Fiber: 1.6g
- Sugar: 1.7g
- Protein: 15.7g

12. QUESO BLANCO DIP

PREPARATION TIME
10'

COOK TIME
15'

SERVING
10

INGREDIENTS

- 2 tablespoons olive oil
- ⅓ cup white onion, chopped finely
- 2 tablespoons jalapeño pepper, minced finely
- 1 pound white American cheese, cut into large pieces
- 8 ounces Monterey Jack cheese, cut into large pieces
- ½ cup half-and-half
- 1/3-½ cup tomato, chopped
- 2 tablespoons fresh cilantro, chopped and divided
- 1 jalapeño pepper, chopped

DIRECTIONS

1. In a medium pan, heat oil over medium-low heat and sauté onion and minced jalapeño pepper for about 2–3 minutes.
2. Add the cheeses and half-and-half and stir to combine.
3. Adjust the heat to low and cook for about 2–3 minutes or until cheeses are melted.
4. Add the tomato pieces and stir to combine.
5. Stir in half of the cilantro and remove from the heat.
6. Serve and garnish with remaining cilantro and chopped jalapeno.

NUTRITIONS

- Calories: 306 kcal
- Net Carbs: 0g
- Total Fat: 25.7g
- Saturated Fat: 13.7g
- Cholesterol: 65mg
- Sodium: 807mg
- Total Carbs: 4.6g
- Fiber: 0.2g
- Sugar: 3.7g
- Protein: 14.1g T

13. STUFFED JALAPENO

PREPARATION TIME
15'

COOK TIME
0

SERVING
10

INGREDIENTS

- 8 ounces cream cheese, softened
- 2 tablespoons fresh chives, minced
- 1 tablespoon pimiento peppers, minced
- ¼ cup mayonnaise
- 26 ounces jalapeño peppers (pickled in a can)

DIRECTIONS

1. In a bowl, add the cream cheese and beat until smooth.
2. Add the mayonnaise, chives, and pimientos, and stir until smooth.
3. Fill each jalapeño pepper with cream cheese mixture.
4. Serve immediately.

NUTRITIONS

- Calories: 123 kcal
- Net Carbs: 0g
- Total Fat: 10.6g
- Saturated Fat: 5.3g
- Cholesterol: 26mg
- Sodium: 1,376mg
- Total Carbs: 5.8g
- Fiber: 2.2g
- Sugar: 2g
- Protein: 2.5g

14. CHEDDAR BISCUITS

PREPARATION TIME
15'

COOK TIME
11'

SERVING
9

INGREDIENTS

- 1½ cups superfine almond flour
- 1 tablespoon organic baking powder
- ½ teaspoon garlic powder
- ½ teaspoon onion powder
- ¼ teaspoon salt
- ½ cup sour cream
- 4 tablespoons unsalted butter, melted
- 2 large organic eggs
- ½ cup cheddar cheese, shredded

DIRECTIONS

1. Preheat your oven to 450°F. Lightly grease 9 cups of a muffin pan.
2. In a large bowl, mix together the almond flour, baking powder, and seasoning.
3. In a small bowl, add the sour cream, butter, and eggs, and beat until smooth.
4. Add the egg mixture into the large bowl of the flour mixture and mix until well combined.
5. Gently, fold in the cheese.
6. Divide the mixture into the prepared muffin cups.
7. Bake for approximately 10–11 minutes or until the tops become golden.
8. Serve warm.

NUTRITIONS

- Calories: 236 kcal
- Net Carbs: 0g
- Total Fat: 21g
- Saturated Fat: 7.2g
- Cholesterol: 67mg
- Sodium: 165mg
- Total Carbs: 5.1g
- Fiber: 2.1g
- Sugar: 0.9g
- Protein: 3.5g

15. CRAB BITES

PREPARATION TIME
15'

COOK TIME
8'

SERVING
8T

INGREDIENTS

- 1 pound canned crabmeat; drained, flaked, and cartilage removed
- 2-2½ cups pork rinds, crushed
- ¾ cup mayonnaise
- 1 large organic egg, beaten
- ⅓ cup celery, chopped
- ⅓ cup green bell pepper, seeded and chopped
- ⅓ cup onion, chopped
- 1 tablespoon fresh parsley, minced
- 2 teaspoons fresh lemon juice
- 1 teaspoon Worcestershire sauce
- ⅛ teaspoon hot pepper sauce
- 1 teaspoon prepared mustard
- 1 tablespoon seafood seasoning
- Ground black pepper, to taste
- 2–4 tablespoons olive oil

DIRECTIONS

1. In a large bowl, add all the ingredients (except for oil) and mix until well combined.
2. Make 8 equal-sized patties from the mixture.
3. In a cast-iron skillet, heat the oil over medium heat and cook the patties for about 4 minutes per side.
4. Serve warm.

NUTRITIONS

- Calories: 277 kcal
- Net Carbs: 0g
- Total Fat: 23.1g
- Saturated Fat: 4.1g
- Cholesterol: 73mg
- Sodium: 686mg
- Total Carbs: 2.2g
- Fiber: 0.3g
- Sugar: 0.6g
- Protein: 13.3g

16. STUFFED MUSHROOMS

 **PREPARATION TIME** 15'

 **COOK TIME** 45'

 **SERVING** 4

INGREDIENTS

- 6 ounces clams
- 1 tablespoon butter, softened
- 1 tablespoon scallion, chopped finely
- ½ teaspoon garlic, minced
- 1 teaspoon dried oregano
- ⅛ teaspoon garlic salt
- ½ cup Italian pork rind
- 1 egg, beaten
- ¼ cup plus 2 tablespoons mozzarella cheese, grated and divided
- 2 tablespoons Parmesan cheese, grated
- 1 tablespoon Romano cheese, grated
- ¼ cup butter, melted
- 8 mushrooms, stems removed
- 2 tablespoons fresh parsley, chopped

DIRECTIONS

1. Preheat your oven to 350°F.
2. Grease a baking dish.
3. Drain the clams, reserving the liquid in a bowl.
4. In a bowl, add the clams, softened butter, scallion, garlic, oregano, and garlic salt, and mix well.
5. Add the reserved clam juice, pork rind, and egg, and mix until well combined.
6. Add 2 tablespoons of mozzarella, parmesan, and romano cheese, and mix well.
7. Arrange the mushrooms onto a platter and stuff the cavity of each with clam mixture.
8. Arrange the mushrooms into the prepared baking dish and drizzle with melted butter.
9. Bake for approximately 35–40 minutes.
10. Remove from the oven and sprinkle the mushrooms with the remaining mozzarella cheese.
11. Bake for approximately 5 minutes or until the cheese is just slightly melted.
12. Garnish with parsley and serve.

NUTRITIONS

- Calories: 331 kcal
- Net Carbs: 7g
- Total Fat: 25.6g
- Saturated Fat: 15.1g
- Cholesterol: 111mg
- Sodium: 644mg
- Total Carbs: 8g
- Fiber: 1g
- Sugar: 2.2g
- Protein: 19.2g

17. BROCCOLI TOTS

PREPARATION TIME
15'

COOK TIME
35'

SERVING
12

INGREDIENTS

- 1 (16-ounce) package frozen chopped broccoli
- 3 large organic eggs
- ½ teaspoon dried oregano
- ½ teaspoon garlic powder
- ⅛ teaspoons cayenne pepper
- ⅛ teaspoons red pepper flakes, crushed
- Salt and freshly ground white pepper, to taste
- 1 cup sharp cheddar cheese, grated
- 1 cup almond flour
- Olive oil cooking spray

DIRECTIONS

1. Preheat your oven to 400°F.
2. Line two baking sheets with lightly greased parchment paper.
3. In a microwave-safe bowl, place the broccoli and microwave covered for about 5 minutes, stir it once halfway through.
4. Drain the broccoli well.
5. In a large bowl, place the eggs, oregano, garlic powder, cayenne pepper, red pepper flakes, salt, and white pepper, and beat until well combined.
6. Add the cooked broccoli, cheddar cheese, and almond flour, and mix until well combined.
7. With slightly wet hands, make 24 equal-sized patties from the mixture.
8. Arrange the patties onto prepared baking sheets in a single layer about 2-inch apart.
9. Lightly spray each patty with the cooking spray.
10. Bake for approximately 15 minutes per side or until it's golden-brown from both sides.
11. Remove from the oven and serve warm.

NUTRITIONS

- Calories: 165 kcal
- Net Carbs: 2.6g
- Total Fat: 7.5g
- Saturated: Fat 0.8g
- Cholesterol: 47mg
- Sodium: 42mg
- Total Carbs: 4.9g
- Fiber: 2.3g
- Sugar: 1.2g
- Protein: 3.2g

PREPARATION TIME
15'

COOK TIME
15'

SERVING
2

INGREDIENTS

- 1 medium onion, cut into ½-inch thick rings
- ½ cup coconut flour
- 1 tablespoon heavy whipping cream
- 2 large organic eggs
- ½ cup Parmesan cheese, grated
- 2 ounces pork rinds, crushed

DIRECTIONS

1. Preheat your oven to 425°F.
2. Arrange a greased rack onto a large baking sheet.
3. Break apart the onion rings and discard inside pieces.
4. In a shallow bowl, place the coconut flour.
5. In a second shallow bowl, add the heavy cream and egg and beat until well combined.
6. In a third shallow bowl, mix together parmesan cheese and pork rinds.
7. Coat onion rings with coconut flour, then dip into the egg mixture and finally, coat with cheese mixture.
8. Repeat the procedure of coating once.
9. Arrange the coated onion rings onto the prepared rack in a single layer.
10. Bake for approximately 15 minutes.
11. Serve warm.

NUTRITIONS

- Calories: 368 kcal
- Net Carbs: 5.3g
- Total Fat: 23.2g
- Saturated Fat: 10.2g
- Cholesterol: 253mg
- Sodium: 801mg
- Total Carbs: 7.7g
- Fiber: 2.4g
- Sugar: 3g
- Protein: 33.8g

19. TUNA CROQUETTES

PREPARATION TIME
15'

COOK TIME
16'

SERVING
4

INGREDIENTS

- 24 ounces canned white tuna, drained
- ¼ cup mayonnaise
- 4 large organic eggs
- 2 tablespoons yellow onion, finely chopped
- 1 scallion, sliced thinly
- 4 garlic cloves, minced
- ¾ cup almond flour
- Salt and freshly ground black pepper, to taste
- ¼ cup olive oil

DIRECTIONS

1. In a large bowl, place the tuna, mayonnaise, eggs, onion, scallion, garlic, almond flour, salt, and black pepper, and mix until well combined.
2. Make 8 equal-sized oblong-shaped patties from the mixture.
3. In a large skillet, heat the olive oil over medium-high heat and fry the croquettes in 2 batches for about 2 to 4 minutes per side.
4. With a slotted spoon, transfer the croquettes onto a paper towel-lined plate to drain completely.
5. Serve warm.

NUTRITIONS

- Calories: 492 kcal
- Net Carbs: 6g
- Total Fat: 30.2g
- Saturated Fat: 5.6g
- Cholesterol: 261mg
- Sodium: 585mg
- Total Carbs: 6.8g
- Fiber: 0.8g
- Sugar: 1.9g
- Protein: 48.1g

20. PARMESAN CHICKEN WINGS

PREPARATION TIME	COOK TIME	SERVING
15'	30'	8

INGREDIENTS

- 3 pounds grass-fed chicken wings
- 1½ tablespoons organic baking powder
- Salt and ground black pepper, to taste
- ¼ cup salted butter
- 4 garlic cloves, minced
- 2 teaspoons dried parsley flakes
- ½ teaspoon red pepper flakes, crushed
- ½ cup Parmesan cheese, grated
- 2 tablespoons fresh parsley, chopped

DIRECTIONS

1. Preheat your oven to 250°F.
2. Arrange a rack in the lower third of the oven.
3. Place a greased rack onto a foil-lined baking sheet.
4. In a bowl, add wings, baking powder, salt, and black pepper, and toss to coat well.
5. Arrange wings over the prepared rack into a baking sheet in a single layer.
6. Bake for approximately 30 minutes.
7. Remove chicken wings from the oven and transfer into a large bowl.
8. In a small frying pan, melt the butter over medium heat and sauté the garlic, dried parsley, and red pepper flakes for about 20 to 30 seconds.
9. Remove from the heat and immediately pour it over the chicken wings.
10. Sprinkle with parmesan cheese and toss to coat well.
11. Garnish with fresh parsley and serve immediately.

NUTRITIONS

- Calories: 397 kcal
- Net Carbs: 1.8g
- Total Fat: 16.9g
- Saturated: Fat 7.7g
- Cholesterol: 171mg
- Sodium: 253mg
- Total Carbs: 1.9g
- Fiber: 0.1g
- Sugar: 0g
- Protein: 51.4g

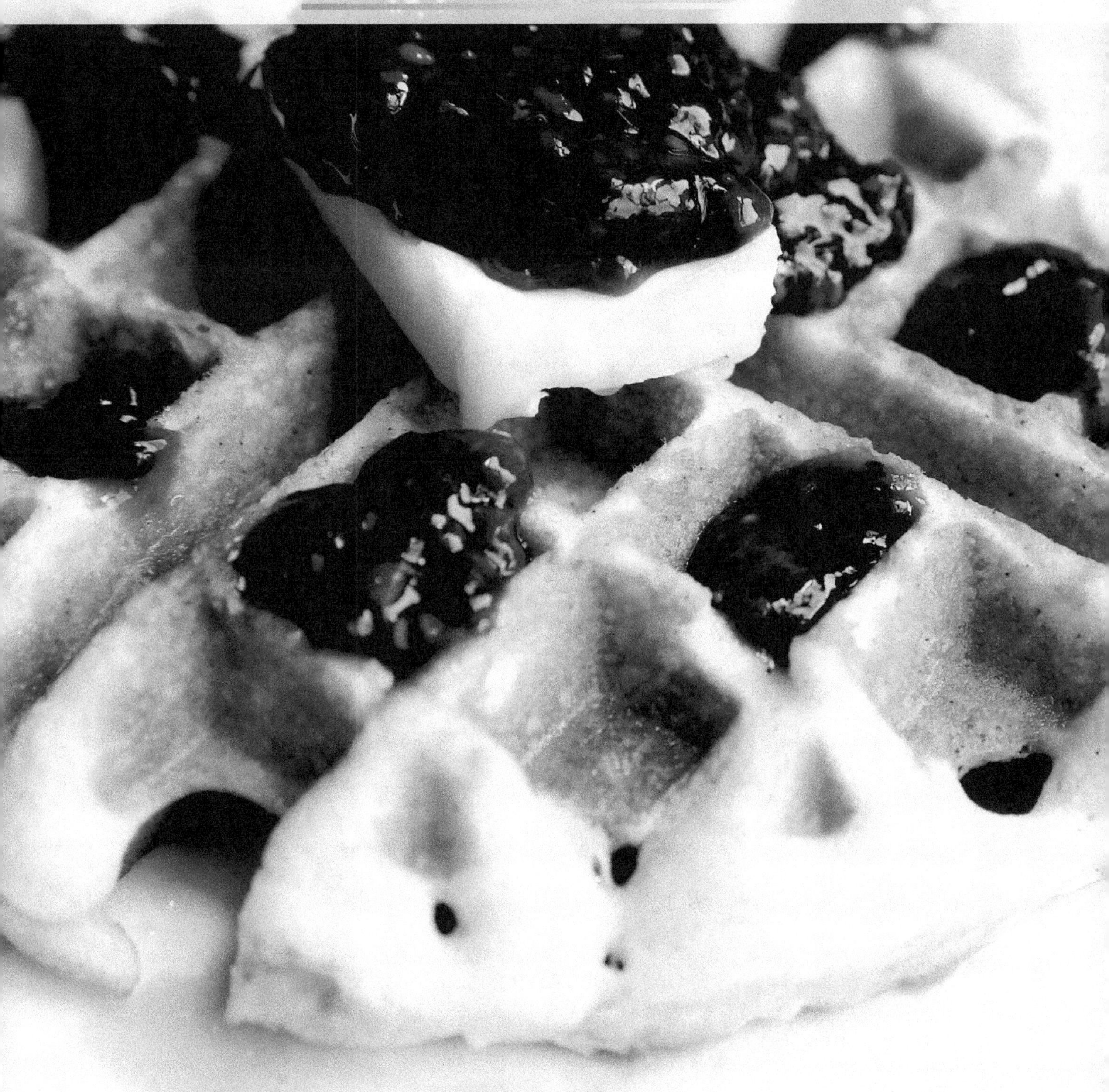

11. DESSERTS

22. BAKED APPLES

PREPARATION TIME
10'

COOK TIME
1 HOUR

SERVING
4

INGREDIENTS

- 4 teaspoon keto-friendly sweetener.
- ¾ teaspoon cinnamon
- ¼ cup chopped pecans
- 4 large Granny Smith apples

DIRECTIONS

1. Set the oven temperature at 375°F. Mix the sweetener with the cinnamon and pecans. Core the apple and add the prepared stuffing.
2. Add enough water into the baking dish to cover the bottom of the apple. Bake them for about 45 minutes to 1 hour.

NUTRITIONS

- Calories: 175 kcal
- Carbohydrates: 16g
- Protein: 6.8g
- Fats: 19.9g

23. KETO CHEESECAKES

PREPARATION TIME
25'

COOK TIME
0

SERVING
9

INGREDIENTS

For the cheesecakes:
- 2 tablespoons butter
- 1 tablespoon caramel syrup; sugar-free
- 3 tablespoons coffee
- 8 ounces cream cheese
- ⅓ cup swerve sweetener
- 3 eggs

For the frosting:
- 8 ounces mascarpone cheese; soft
- 3 tablespoons caramel syrup; sugar-free
- 2 tablespoons swerve
- 3 tablespoons butter

DIRECTIONS

1. In your blender, mix the cream cheese with eggs, 2 tablespoons of butter, coffee, 1 tablespoon caramel syrup, and ⅓ cup swerve. Blend very well.
2. Spoon this into a cupcakes pan, introduce it in the oven at 350 °F and bake for 15 minutes
3. Leave aside to cool down and then keep in the freezer for 3 hours
4. Meanwhile, in a bowl, mix 3 tablespoons butter with 3 tablespoons caramel syrup, 2 tablespoons swerve, and mascarpone cheese and blend well.
5. Spoon this over the cheesecakes and serve them.

NUTRITIONS

- Calories: 478.2 kcal
- Total Fat: 47.8g
- Cholesterol: 140.4mg
- Sodium: 270.7mg
- Potassium: 233.7mg
- Total Carbohydrate: 9.4g
- Protein: 9.2g

24. KETO BROWNIES

PREPARATION TIME
30'

COOK TIME
0

SERVING
12

INGREDIENTS

- 6 ounces coconut oil; melted
- 4 ounces cream cheese
- 5 tablespoons swerve sweetener
- 6 eggs
- 2 teaspoons vanilla
- 3 ounces of cocoa powder
- ½ teaspoon baking powder

DIRECTIONS

1. In a blender, mix the eggs with coconut oil, cocoa powder, baking powder, vanilla, cream cheese, and swerve. Stir using a mixer.
2. Pour this into a lined baking dish, introduce it in the oven at 350°F and bake for 20 minutes
3. Slice into rectangle pieces when it gets cold and serve

NUTRITIONS

- Calories: 183.7 kcal
- Total Fat: 16.6g
- Cholesterol: 20.7mg
- Sodium: 36.3mg
- Potassium: 21.6mg
- Total Carbohydrate: 4.9g
- Protein: 1.4g

KETO DIET COOKBOOK FOR WOMEN OVER 50

25. RASPBERRY AND COCONUT

PREPARATION TIME
15'

COOK TIME
0

SERVING
12

INGREDIENTS

- ¼ cup swerve sweetener
- ½ cup coconut oil
- ½ cup raspberries, dried
- ½ cup coconut; shredded
- ½ cup coconut butter

DIRECTIONS

1. In your food processor, blend the dried berries very well.
2. Heat a pan with the butter over medium heat.
3. Add the oil, coconut and swerve; stir and cook for 5 minutes
4. Pour half of this into a lined baking pan and spread well.
5. Add raspberry powder and also spread.
6. Top with the rest of the butter mix, spread and keep in the fridge for a while
7. Cut into pieces and serve

NUTRITIONS

- Carbohydrates: 45g
- Sugar: 30g
- Fat: 42g
- Protein: 8g
- Cholesterol: 0mg

26. CHOCOLATE PUDDING DELIGHT

PREPARATION TIME
52'

COOK TIME
0

SERVING
2

INGREDIENTS

- ½ teaspoon stevia powder
- 2 tablespoons cocoa powder
- 2 tablespoons water
- 1 tablespoon gelatin
- 1 cup of coconut milk
- 2 tablespoons maple syrup

DIRECTIONS

1. Heat a pan with the coconut milk over medium heat; add stevia and cocoa powder and mix well.
2. In a bowl, mix the gelatin with water; stir well and add to the pan.
3. Stir well, add the maple syrup, whisk again, divide into ramekins and keep in the fridge for 45 minutes. Serve cold.

NUTRITIONS

- Calories: 221.2 kcal
- Total Fat: 13.6g
- Cholesterol: 9.8mg
- Sodium: 250.3mg
- Potassium: 86.7mg
- Total Carbohydrate: 22.7g
- Protein: 3.4g

27. PEANUT BUTTER FUDGE

PREPARATION TIME
2 HOURS 12'

COOK TIME
0

SERVING
12'

INGREDIENTS

- 1 cup peanut butter; unsweetened
- 1 cup coconut oil
- ¼ cup almond milk
- 2 teaspoons vanilla stevia
- A pinch of salt

For the topping:
- 2 tablespoons swerve sweetener
- ¼ cup cocoa powder
- 2 tablespoons melted coconut oil

DIRECTIONS

1. In a heatproof bowl, mix the peanut butter with 1 cup coconut oil; stir and heat up in your microwave until it melts
2. Add a pinch of salt, almond milk, and stevia; stir everything well and pour into a lined loaf pan.
3. Keep in the fridge for 2 hours and then slice it.
4. In a bowl, mix 2 tablespoons of melted coconut oil with cocoa powder, swerve and stir very well.
5. Drizzle the sauce over your peanut butter fudge and serve

NUTRITIONS

- Calories: 85 kcal
- Fat: 4.7g
- Saturated Fat: 2.7g
- Protein: 0.5g

28. CINNAMON STREUSEL EGG LOAF

PREPARATION TIME
10'

COOK TIME
15'

SERVING
2

INGREDIENTS

- 2 tablespoons almond flour
- 1 tablespoons butter, softened
- ½ tablespoons grated butter, chilled
- 1 egg
- 1-ounce cream cheese

Others:
- ½ teaspoon cinnamon, divided
- 1 tablespoons erythritol sweetener, divided
- ¼ teaspoon vanilla extract, unsweetened

DIRECTIONS

1. Turn on the oven, then set it to 350°F and let it preheat.
2. Meanwhile, crack the egg in a small bowl; add cream cheese, softened butter, ¼ tsp. cinnamon, ½ tablespoon sweetener, and vanilla and whisk until well combined.
3. Divide the egg batter between two silicone muffins and then bake for 7 minutes.
4. Meanwhile, prepare the streusel and for this, place flour in a small bowl, add the remaining ingredients, and stir until well mixed.
5. When egg loaves have baked, sprinkle streusel on top and then and continue baking for 7 minutes.
6. When done, remove loaves from the cups, let them cool for 5 minutes and then serve and enjoy!

NUTRITIONS

- Calories: 152 kcal
- Fats: 14.8g
- Protein: 4.1g
- Net Carbohydrates: 1.3g
- Fiber: 0.9g

29. SNICKERDOODLE MUFFINS

 **PREPARATION TIME** 10'

 **COOK TIME** 12'

 **SERVING** 2

INGREDIENTS

- 6 ⅔ tablespoons coconut flour
- ½ egg
- 1 tablespoons butter, unsalted and melted
- 1 ⅓ tablespoons whipping cream
- 1 tablespoon almond milk, unsweetened

Others:
- 1 ⅓ tablespoons erythritol sweetener and more for topping
- ¼ teaspoon baking powder
- ¼ teaspoon ground cinnamon and more for topping
- ¼ teaspoon vanilla extract, unsweetened

DIRECTIONS

1. Turn on the oven, then set it to 350 °F and let it preheat.
2. Meanwhile, take a medium bowl, place flour in it, and add the cinnamon and baking powder. Stir until well combined.
3. Take a separate bowl, place the half egg in it, add butter, sour cream, milk, and vanilla, and whisk until well blended.
4. Whisk in flour mixture until a smooth batter is obtained, divide the batter evenly between two silicone muffin cups, and then sprinkle cinnamon and sweetener on top.
5. Bake the muffins for 10 to 12 minutes until firm and the top has turned golden brown and then serve and enjoy!

NUTRITIONS

- Calories: 241 kcal
- Fats: 21g
- Protein: 7g
- Net Carbohydrates: 3g
- Fiber: 3g

30. YOGURT AND STRAWBERRY BOWL

PREPARATION TIME	**COOK TIME**	**SERVING**
5'	0	2

INGREDIENTS

- 3 ounces mixed berries
- 1 tablespoon chopped almonds
- 1 tablespoon chopped walnuts
- 4 ounces yogurt

DIRECTIONS

1. Divide the yogurt between two bowls, top with berries and then sprinkle with almonds and walnuts.
2. Serve and enjoy!

NUTRITIONS

- Calories: 165 kcal
- Fats: 11.2g
- Protein: 9.3g
- Net Carbohydrates: 2.5g
- Fiber: 1.8g

31. SWEET CINNAMON MUFFIN

PREPARATION TIME
5'

COOK TIME
2'

SERVING
2

INGREDIENTS

- 4 teaspoon coconut flour
- 2 teaspoon cinnamon
- 2 teaspoon erythritol sweetener
- 1/16 teaspoon baking soda
- 2 eggs

DIRECTIONS

1. Take a medium bowl, place all the ingredients in it, and whisk until well combined.
2. Take two ramekins, grease them with oil, distribute the prepared batter in it and then microwave for 1 minute and 45 seconds until done.
3. When done, take out muffin from the ramekin, cut it in half, and then serve and enjoy!

NUTRITIONS

- Calories: 101 kcal
- Fats: 6.5g
- Protein: 7.6g
- Net Carbohydrates: 0.5g
- Fiber: 1.7g

32. NUTTY MUFFINS

PREPARATION TIME
5'

COOK TIME
5'

SERVING
2

INGREDIENTS

- 4 teaspoons coconut flour
- 1/16 teaspoon baking soda
- 1 teaspoon erythritol sweetener
- 2 eggs
- 2 teaspoons almond butter, unsalted

DIRECTIONS

1. Take a medium bowl, place all the ingredients in it, and whisk until well combined.
2. Take two ramekins, grease them with oil, distribute the prepared batter in it and then microwave for 1 minute and 45 seconds until done.
3. When done, take out muffin from the ramekin, cut it in half, and then serve and enjoy!

NUTRITIONS

- Calories: 131 kcal
- Fats: 8.6g
- Protein: 8.4g
- Net Carbohydrates: 2.3g
- Fiber: 2.2g

33. PUMPKIN AND CREAM CHEESE CUP

 **PREPARATION TIME**
10'

 **COOK TIME**
12'

 **SERVING**
2

INGREDIENTS

- 4 tablespoons almond flour
- 1 ⅓ tablespoon coconut flour
- 2 tablespoon pumpkin puree
- 2 ⅔ tablespoon cream cheese, softened
- ½ egg
- ⅔ tablespoon butter, unsalted
- ¼ teaspoon pumpkin spice
- ⅔ teaspoon baking powder
- 2 tablespoon erythritol sweetener

DIRECTIONS

1. Turn on the oven, then set it to 350 °F and let it preheat.
2. Take a medium bowl, place the butter and 1 ½ tablespoon sweetener in it, and then beat until it's fluffy.
3. Beat in the egg and then beat in the pumpkin puree until well combined.
4. Take a medium bowl, place the flours in it, stir in pumpkin spice, baking powder until mixed, stir this mixture into the butter mixture and then distribute it into two silicone muffin cups.
5. Take a medium bowl, place cream cheese in it, and stir in the remaining sweetener until well combined.
6. Divide the cream cheese mixture into the silicone muffin cups, swirl the batter and cream cheese mixture by using a toothpick and then bake for 10 to 12 minutes until muffins have turned firm.
7. Serve and enjoy!

NUTRITIONS

- Calories: 261 kcal
- Fats: 23g
- Protein: 7g
- Net Carbohydrates: 2g
- Fiber: 4g

34. BERRIES IN YOGURT CREAM

PREPARATION TIME
1 H 5'

COOK TIME
0

SERVING
2

INGREDIENTS

- 1-ounce blackberries
- 1-ounce raspberry
- 2 tablespoons erythritol sweetener
- 4 ounces yogurt
- 4 ounces whipping cream

DIRECTIONS

1. Take a medium bowl, place the yogurt in it, and then whisk until it's creamy.
2. Sprinkle the sweetener over the yogurt mixture, don't stir, cover the bowl with a lid, and then refrigerate for 1 hour.
3. When ready to serve, stir the yogurt mixture, divide it evenly between two bowls, top with berries, and then serve and enjoy!

NUTRITIONS

- Calories: 245 kcal
- Fats: 22g
- Protein: 4.2g
- Net Carbohydrates: 5g
- Fiber: 1.7g

35. PUMPKIN PIE MUG CAKE

PREPARATION TIME
5'

COOK TIME
2'

SERVING
2

INGREDIENTS

- 2 tablespoons coconut flour
- 1 teaspoon sour cream
- 2 tablespoons whipping cream
- 2 eggs
- ¼ cup pumpkin puree

Others:
- 2 tablespoons erythritol sweetener
- ⅓ teaspoon cinnamon
- ¼ teaspoon baking soda

DIRECTIONS

1. Take a small bowl, place the cream in it, and then beat in the sweetener until well combined.
2. Cover the bowl, let it chill in the refrigerator for 30 minutes, then beat in the eggs and pumpkin puree and stir in remaining ingredients until incorporated and smooth.
3. Divide the batter between two coffee mugs greased with oil and then microwave for 2 minutes until thoroughly cooked.
4. Serve and enjoy!

NUTRITIONS

- Calories: 181 kcal
- Fats: 12.1g
- Protein: 8.8g
- Net Carbohydrates: 4.6g
- Fiber: 3.3g

36. CHOCOLATE AND STRAWBERRY CREPE

PREPARATION TIME	**COOK TIME**	**SERVING**
5'	5'	2

INGREDIENTS

- 1 ⅓ tablespoon coconut flour
- 1 teaspoon of cocoa powder
- ¼ teaspoon flaxseed
- 1 egg
- 2 ¾ tablespoons coconut milk, unsweetened
- 2 teaspoons avocado oil
- ⅛ teaspoon baking powder
- 2 ounces strawberry, sliced

DIRECTIONS

1. Take a medium bowl, place the flour in it, and then stir in the cocoa powder, baking powder, and flaxseed in it until well mixed.
2. Add the egg and milk and then whisk until smooth.
3. Take a medium skillet pan, place it over medium heat, add 1 teaspoon of oil and when hot, pour in half of the batter, spread it evenly, and then cook for 1 minute per side until firm.
4. Transfer crepe to a plate, add remaining oil, and cook another crepe by using the remaining batter.
5. When done, fill crepes with strawberries, fold them and then serve and enjoy!

NUTRITIONS

- Calories: 120 kcal
- Fats: 8.5g
- Protein: 4.4g
- Carbohydrates: 2.8g
- Fiber: 2.7g

37. BANANA PANCAKES

PREPARATION TIME
10'

COOK TIME
15'

SERVING
3

INGREDIENTS

- Butter
- 2 Bananas
- 4 Eggs
- 1 teaspoon Cinnamon
- 1 teaspoon Baking powder (Optional)

DIRECTIONS

1. Combine each of the fixings. Melt a portion of the butter in a skillet using the medium temperature setting.
2. Prepare the pancakes 1-2 minutes per side. Cook them with the lid on for the first part of the cooking cycle for a fluffier pancake.
3. Serve plain or with your favorite garnishes such as a dollop of coconut cream or fresh berries.

NUTRITIONS

- Calories: 157 kcal
- Carbohydrates: 6.8g
- Total Fat: 7g

38. COCONUT MACADAMIA BARS

PREPARATION TIME
15'

COOK TIME
REFRIGERATION

SERVING
6

INGREDIENTS

- ½ cup macadamia nuts
- 6 tablespoons unsweetened coconut, shredded
- ½ cup almond butter
- 20 stevia drops, preferably SweetLeaf
- ¼ cup coconut oil

DIRECTIONS

1. Crush the macadamia nuts using your hands or in a food processor.
2. Combine the coconut oil with the shredded coconut and almond butter in a large-sized mixing bowl. Add the stevia drops and chopped macadamia nuts.
3. Thoroughly mix and pour the prepared batter into a 9x9" baking dish lined with parchment paper.
4. Refrigerate overnight
5. Slice into desired pieces. Serve and enjoy.

NUTRITIONS

- Calories: 324 kcal
- Total Fat: 32g
- Saturated Fat: 13g
- Total Carbohydrates: 5g
- Dietary Fiber: 4g
- Sugars: 1.8g
- Protein: 5.6g

39. MACADAMIA CHOCOLATE FAT BOMB

PREPARATION TIME
15'

COOK TIME
REFRIGERATION

SERVING
6

INGREDIENTS

- 2 ounces cocoa butter
- 4 ounces macadamias, chopped
- 2 tablespoons swerve
- ¼ cup coconut oil or heavy cream
- 2 tablespoons cocoa powder, unsweetened

DIRECTIONS

1. Fill a large saucepan half full with boiling water. Place a small-sized saucepan over the large saucepan with the boiling water and melt the cocoa butter in it.
2. Once melted add in the cocoa powder and then add the swerve
3. Mix well until the entire ingredients are completely melted and well blended.
4. Add in the macadamias
5. Give everything a good stir.
6. Now, add the cream or coconut oil
7. Mix well (bringing it to the temperature again). Pour the prepared mixture into paper candy cups or molds filling them evenly. Let cool for a couple of minutes at room temperature and then place them in a refrigerator. Let chill until it hardens. Serve and enjoy.

NUTRITIONS

- Calories: 267 kcal
- Total Fat: 28g
- Saturated Fat: 15g
- Total Carbohydrates: 3g
- Dietary Fiber: 2g
- Sugars: 0.9g
- Protein: 3g

40. BLACKBERRY AND COCONUT FLOUR CUPCAKE

PREPARATION TIME
5'

COOK TIME
15'

SERVING
2

INGREDIENTS

- 3 ¼ tablespoons coconut flour
- ⅓ cup whipping cream
- 1 tablespoon cream cheese
- 1 ½ egg
- 1-ounce blackberry
- 2 ⅔ tablespoons butter, unsalted, chopped
- 5 ⅓ tablespoons erythritol sweetener
- ⅔ teaspoon baking powder
- ⅓ teaspoon vanilla extract, unsweetened

DIRECTIONS

1. Take a small bowl, place the butter in it, and add cream, and then microwave for 30 to 60 seconds until it melts, stirring every 20 seconds.
2. Then add the cream cheese, cream, vanilla, and erythritol, whisk until smooth. Whisk in the coconut flour and baking powder until incorporated and then add in the berries.
3. Distribute the mixture evenly between four muffin cups, then bake for 12 to 15 minutes until firm.
4. Serve and enjoy!

NUTRITIONS

- Calorie: 420 kcal
- Fats: 38.2g
- Protein: 9.4g
- Net Carbohydrates: 5.7g
- Fiber: 4.8g

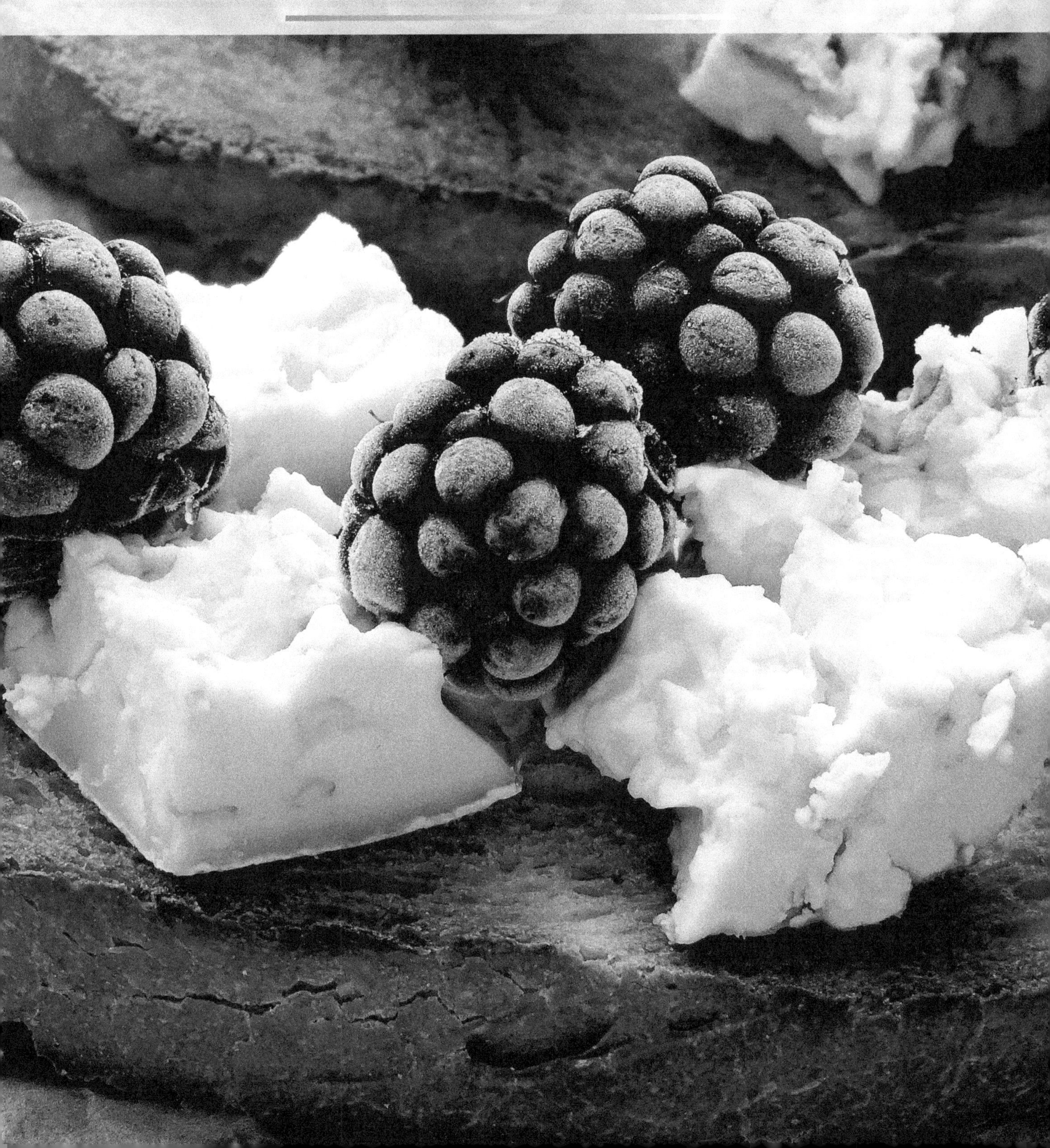

12. MORE KETO RECIPES

1. CREAM CHEESE PANCAKE

PREPARATION TIME
5'

COOK TIME
7'

SERVING
1

INGREDIENTS

- ½ to 1 packet of Stevia
- 1 tablespoon coconut flour
- ½ teaspoon cinnamon
- 2 eggs
- 2 ounces cream cheese

DIRECTIONS

1. Combine well all of the ingredients in a bowl until the mixture is smooth, then heat a skillet over medium-high heat and add in the coconut oil.
2. Add a scoop of the batter into the heated pan and cook for about 2 minutes on both sides. Repeat the same procedure for the remaining batter.
3. Top the pancakes with sugar-free maple syrup.

NUTRITIONS

- Calories: 365 kcal
- Fat: 19g
- Carbs: 8g
- Protein: 17g

2. GREEK STYLE LAMB CHOPS

PREPARATION TIME
15'

COOK TIME
10 - 15'

SERVING
2

INGREDIENTS

- 1 tablespoon black pepper
- 1 tablespoon dried oregano
- 1 tablespoon minced garlic
- 2 tablespoons lemon juice
- 2 teaspoons oil
- 2 teaspoons salt
- 8 pcs lamb loin chops, around 4 ounces

DIRECTIONS

1. In a big bowl or dish, combine the black pepper, salt, minced garlic, lemon juice, and oregano. Then rub it equally on all sides of the lamb chops.
2. Then place a skillet on high heat. After a minute, coat the skillet with cooking spray and place the lamb chops. Sear the lamb chops for a minute on each side.
3. Lower the heat to medium, continue cooking the lamb chops for 2-3 minutes per side or until the desired doneness is reached. Let it cool.

NUTRITIONS

- Calories: 270 kcal
- Fat: 17g
- Carbs: 2g
- Protein: 27g

3. KETO-APPROVED BEEF RAGU

PREPARATION TIME
15'

COOK TIME
15'

SERVING
2

INGREDIENTS

- ¼ pound ground beef
- 1 teaspoon salt
- 2 large zucchinis, cut into noodle strips
- 1 tablespoon ghee or butter
- 4 tablespoons fresh parsley, chopped

DIRECTIONS

1. Heat the ghee in a skillet under medium flame and cook the ground beef until thoroughly cooked, for around 5 minutes.
2. Add the packaged pesto sauce and season with salt. Add the chopped parsley and cook for three more minutes. Set aside.
3. In the same saucepan, place the zucchini noodles and cook for 5 minutes. Turn off the heat then add the cooked meat. Mix well and let it cool.

NUTRITIONS

- Calories: 176 kcal
- Fat: 5g
- Carbs: 4g
- Protein: 27g

4. BACON-WRAPPED ROASTED ASPARAGUS

 **PREPARATION TIME**
10'

 **COOK TIME**
15'

 **SERVING**
2

INGREDIENTS

- 16 asparagus spear, ends trimmed
- 16 pieces bacon
- 2 tablespoons extra-virgin olive oil
- Salt and pepper to taste

DIRECTIONS

1. Preheat the oven to 400°F.
2. Line a baking sheet with aluminum foil or parchment paper.
3. Place the dry asparagus and place it on the baking sheet. Drizzle with the olive oil and toss to coat. Add salt and pepper to taste.
4. Wrap each spear with the bacon. Bake for 10 more minutes. Let it cool.

NUTRITIONS

- Calories: 71 kcal
- Fat: 4g
- Carbs: 1g
- Protein: 6g

5. KETO REUBEN SKILLET

PREPARATION TIME

5'

COOK TIME

10'

SERVING

2

INGREDIENTS

- 1 dill pickle
- 4 ounces Swiss cheese
- ½ cup mayonnaise
- 1 tablespoon Dijon mustard
- 9 ounces drained sauerkraut
- 10 ounces corned beef
- 2 tablespoons butter

DIRECTIONS

1. Put some butter in a skillet on medium to low heat.
2. Put in the beef and carefully fry it, then dry the sauerkraut.
3. Remove as much liquid from it and place it evenly in a skillet.
4. Put some scoops of mustard in the skillet with the sauerkraut, then put in Swiss cheese and cook until the cheese begins to melt.
5. Cover the pan to make the mixture cook faster. Serve with more mustard and dill pickles.

NUTRITIONS

- Calories: 1104 kcal
- Fat: 93g
- Carbs: 3g
- Protein: 58g

6. CAULI MAC AND CHEESE

 **PREPARATION TIME**
15'

 **COOK TIME**
20'

 **SERVING**
4

INGREDIENTS

- 1 head cauliflower, cut into florets
- 2 tablespoons ghee, melted
- Salt and black pepper, to taste
- ½ cup crème fraîche
- ½ cup half-and-half
- 1 cup cream cheese
- ½ teaspoon turmeric powder
- 1 teaspoon garlic paste
- ½ teaspoon onion flakes

DIRECTIONS

1. Set the oven to 450°F. Grease a baking sheet with cooking spray.
2. Mix the cauliflower florets with melted ghee, salt, and pepper. Arrange on the baking sheet and roast for 15 minutes. In a saucepan over medium heat, pour the remaining ingredients and heat through, stirring frequently. Reduce heat to low and simmer for 2-3 minutes until thickened.
3. Coat the cauliflower florets in the cheese sauce and serve immediately in serving bowls.

NUTRITIONS

- Calories: 237 kcal
- Fat: 15g
- Carbs: 11g
- Protein: 16g

7. CHEESE & PUMPKIN CHICKEN MEATBALLS

PREPARATION TIME
15'

COOK TIME
30'

SERVING
5

INGREDIENTS

- 1 egg, beaten
- 1 pound ground chicken
- 1 carrot, grated
- 2 garlic cloves, minced
- 1 onion, chopped
- 1 tablespoon Italian mixed herbs
- Salt and black pepper, to taste
- 2 tablespoon olive oil
- 1 cup cheddar cheese, shredded

DIRECTIONS

1. Set the oven to 360°F. Combine all ingredients, excluding the cheese.
2. Form meatballs from the mixture; set them on a parchment-lined baking sheet. Bake for 25 minutes, flipping them once.
3. Spread the cheese over the balls and bake for 7 more minutes or until all cheese melts.

NUTRITIONS

- Calories: 140 kcal
- Fat: 8g
- Carbs: 2g
- Protein: 16g

8. CHEESE, HAM AND EGG MUFFINS

PREPARATION TIME
20'

COOK TIME
15'

SERVING
6-8

INGREDIENTS

- 24 slices smoked ham
- 6 eggs, beaten
- Salt and black pepper, to taste
- ¼ cup fresh parsley, chopped
- ¼ cup ricotta cheese
- ¼ cup Brie, chopped

DIRECTIONS

1. Set the oven to 390°F.
2. Line 2 slices of smoked ham to each muffin cup to circle each mold.
3. In a mixing bowl, mix the rest of the ingredients. Fill ¾ of the ham lined muffin cup with the egg/cheese mixture.
4. Bake for 15 minutes. Serve warm.

NUTRITIONS

- Calories: 108 kcal
- Fat: 6g
- Carbs: 1g
- Protein: 10g

9. BEEF AND KALE PAN

PREPARATION TIME
10'

COOK TIME
20'

SERVING
4

INGREDIENTS

- 1 pound beef stew meat, cubed
- 1 tablespoon olive oil
- 1 cup kale, torn
- 1 teaspoon chili powder
- 1 teaspoon rosemary, dried
- 1 red onion, chopped
- 2 garlic cloves, minced
- 1 cup beef stock
- ½ teaspoon sweet paprika
- 1 tablespoon cilantro, chopped

DIRECTIONS

1. Make sure that you heat the pan; add the onion and the garlic, stir and sauté for 2 minutes.
2. Add the meat and brown it for 5 minutes.
3. Add the rest of the ingredients, bring to a simmer then cook over medium heat for 13 more minutes.
4. Divide the mix between plates and serve for lunch.

NUTRITIONS

- Calories: 160 kcal
- Fat: 10g
- Carbs: 1g
- Protein: 12g

10. CHILI EGG PICKLES

PREPARATION TIME
15'

COOK TIME
20'

SERVING
4

INGREDIENTS

- 10 eggs
- ½ cup onions, sliced
- 3 cardamom pods
- 1 tablespoon chili powder
- 1 teaspoon yellow seeds
- 2 garlic cloves, sliced
- 1 cup vinegar
- 1 ¼ cups water
- 1 tablespoon salt

DIRECTIONS

1. Boil the eggs in salted water until hard-cooked, for about 10 minutes, rinse under cold running water; peel and discard the shell.
2. Place the peeled eggs into a large jar. Set a pan over medium heat. Stir in all remaining ingredients and bring to a rapid boil.
3. Reduce heat to low; allow simmering for 6 minutes. Spoon this mixture into the jar. Refrigerate for 2 to 3 weeks.

NUTRITIONS

- Calories: 127 kcal
- Fat: 8g
- Carbs: 3g
- Protein: 12g

11. GINGERY TUNA MOUSSE

PREPARATION TIME
15'

COOK TIME
15'

SERVING
3

INGREDIENTS

- 1 ½ teaspoon gelatin, powdered
- 2 ounces ricotta cheese
- 1 teaspoon mustard
- ¼ cup onions, chopped
- ½ teaspoon salt
- ⅓ teaspoon ginger, grated
- 3 tablespoons water
- 3 tablespoons mayonnaise
- 3 ounces canned tuna, flaked
- 1 garlic clove, minced
- ¼ teaspoon black pepper

DIRECTIONS

1. Mix the gelatin in water; let sit for 10 minutes. Set a pan over medium heat and warm the ricotta cheese, place in the gelatin and mix to blend well. Let the mixture cool.
2. Place in the other ingredients and stir.
3. Split the mixture among 5 mousse molds and refrigerate overnight. Serve by inverting the molds over a serving platter.

NUTRITIONS

- Calories: 109 kcal
- Fat: 6g
- Carbs: 0g
- Protein: 18g

12. CREAMY CHEDDAR DEVILED EGGS

PREPARATION TIME
10'

COOK TIME
15'

SERVING
10

INGREDIENTS

- 10 eggs
- ¼ cup mayonnaise
- 1 tablespoon tomato paste
- 2 tablespoons celery, chopped
- 2 tablespoons carrot, chopped
- 2 tablespoons chives, minced
- 2 tablespoons cheddar cheese, grated
- Salt and black pepper, to taste

DIRECTIONS

1. Place the eggs in a pot and fill with water by about 1 inch. Bring the eggs to a boil over high heat, then reduce the heat to medium and simmer for 10 minutes.
2. Remove and rinse under running water until cooled. Peel and discard the shell.
3. Slice each egg in half lengthwise and get rid of the yolks. Mix the yolks with the rest of the ingredients.
4. Split the mixture amongst the egg whites and set deviled eggs on a plate to serve.

NUTRITIONS

- Calories: 120 kcal
- Fat: 11g
- Carbs: 1g
- Protein: 6g

13. DARK CHOCOLATE COVERED WALNUTS

 **PREPARATION TIME** 15'

 **COOK TIME** 10'

 **SERVING** 6

INGREDIENTS

- 2 cups shelled walnuts
- ½ cup unsweetened chocolate, chopped
- ¼ cup powdered Stevia or any other natural sweetener
- 3 tablespoons walnut oil
- ½ teaspoon vanilla extract
- 1 tablespoon unsweetened cocoa powder

DIRECTIONS

1. Take a pan; combine the chocolate, powdered Swerve, and walnut oil on low heat.
2. Stir well until melted and smooth. Now add in the vanilla extract and cocoa powder until smooth. Let the mixture cool for 5 minutes to thicken.
3. Now dip the walnuts in the chocolate mixture, do the same with all the walnuts. Place them on a baking sheet and chill in the freezer until firm. They can be stored in an airtight container for a few days.

NUTRITIONS

- Calories: 160 kcal
- Fat: 11g
- Carbs: 15g
- Protein: 2g

14. HOMEMADE GRAHAM CRACKERS

PREPARATION TIME
20'

COOK TIME
60'

SERVING
10

INGREDIENTS

- 1½ cups almond flour
- 1⅓ cups graham flour
- 1 teaspoon baking soda
- ½ teaspoon salt
- 2 tablespoons unsalted butter
- ⅔ cups dark brown sugar
- Vanilla extract
- 1 egg

DIRECTIONS

1. Preheat the oven to 180°C. In a bowl, beat the graham flour, almond flour, sweetener, baking powder and salt.
2. Blend in the vanilla extract, egg and melted butter until dough becomes a mixture. Make rough rectangles of the dough.
3. Use a knife or a pizza wheel to cut into squares of about 2x2 inches. Transfer the pieces to a baking sheet. Bake for 20 to 30 minutes, until golden brown.
4. Take them out and let them cool again. Enjoy crispy crackers.

NUTRITIONS

- Calories: 31 kcal
- Fat: 0g
- Carbs: 7g
- Protein: 1g

15. CHOCOLATE COCONUT KETO SMOOTHIE BOWL

PREPARATION TIME	**COOK TIME**	**SERVING**
15'	10'	3-6

INGREDIENTS

- ⅓ cup vanilla protein powder
- ½ cup almond milk
- 1 tablespoon cocoa powder
- 1 tablespoon coconut oil
- Sweetener
- 3 cups crushed ice
- ⅛ teaspoon xanthan gum
- ½ cup raspberries
- ¼ cup walnuts
- 2 tablespoons pomegranate

DIRECTIONS

1. Take a blender, pour the almond milk, protein powder, cocoa powder, sweetener and ice, and blend the ingredients well.
2. Now add the coconut oil, xanthan gum and blend until it increases in volume. Pour it into a bowl, add fruits and nuts and serve.

NUTRITIONS

- Calories: 141 kcal
- Fat: 9g
- Carbs: 5g
- Protein: 14g

16. SPICED JALAPEÑO BITES WITH TOMATO

PREPARATION TIME	COOK TIME	SERVING
10'	0	4

INGREDIENTS

- 1 cup turkey ham, chopped
- ¼ jalapeño pepper, minced
- ¼ cup mayonnaise
- ⅓ tablespoon Dijon mustard
- 4 tomatoes, sliced
- Salt and black pepper, to taste
- 1 tablespoon parsley, chopped

DIRECTIONS

1. In a bowl, mix the turkey ham, jalapeño pepper, mayo, mustard, salt, and pepper.
2. Spread out the tomato slices on four serving plates, and then top each plate with a spoonful of the turkey ham mixture.
3. Serve garnished with chopped parsley.

NUTRITIONS

- Calories: 250 kcal
- Fat: 14.1g
- Fiber: 3.7g
- Carbohydrates: 4.1g
- Protein: 18.9g

17. COCONUT CRAB CAKES

PREPARATION TIME
20'

COOK TIME
25'

SERVING
4

INGREDIENTS

- 1 tablespoon garlic, minced
- 2 pasteurized eggs
- 2 teaspoons coconut oil
- ¾ cup coconut flakes
- ¾ cup chopped spinach
- ¼ pound crabmeat
- ¼ cup chopped leek
- ½ cup extra virgin olive oil
- ½ teaspoon pepper
- ¼ onion, diced
- Salt

DIRECTIONS

1. Pour the crabmeat into a bowl, then add in the coconut flakes and mix well.
2. Whisk eggs in a bowl, and then mix in the leek and spinach.
3. Season the egg mixture with pepper, two pinches of salt, and garlic.
4. Then, pour the eggs into the crab and stir well.
5. Preheat a pan, heat the extra virgin olive oil, and fry the crab evenly from each side until golden brown. Remove from the pan and serve hot.

NUTRITIONS

- Calories: 254 kcal
- Fat: 9.5g
- Fiber: 5.4g
- Carbohydrates: 4.1g
- Protein: 8.9g

18. TUNA BURGERS

PREPARATION TIME
15'

COOK TIME
10'

SERVING
2

INGREDIENTS

- 1 (15-ounce) can water-packed tuna, drained
- ½ celery stalk, chopped
- 2 tablespoon fresh parsley, chopped
- 1 teaspoon fresh dill, chopped
- 2 tablespoons walnuts, chopped
- 2 tablespoons mayonnaise
- 1 organic egg, beaten
- 1 tablespoon butter
- 3 cups lettuce

DIRECTIONS

1. For burgers: Add all ingredients (except the butter and lettuce) in a bowl and mix until well combined.
2. Make two equal-sized patties from the mixture.
3. Melt some butter and cook the patties for about 2–3 minutes.
4. Carefully flip the side and cook for about 2–3 minutes.
5. Divide the lettuce onto serving plates.
6. Top each plate with one burger and serve.

NUTRITIONS

- Calories: 267 kcal
- Fat: 12.5g
- Fiber: 9.4g
- Carbohydrates: 3.8g
- Protein: 11.5g

19. CREAMED SPINACH

PREPARATION TIME
10'

COOK TIME
15'

SERVING
4

INGREDIENTS

- 2 tablespoons unsalted butter
- 1 small yellow onion, chopped
- 1 cup cream cheese, softened
- 2 (10-ounce) packages frozen spinach, thawed and squeezed dry
- 2–3 tablespoons water
- Salt and ground black pepper, as required
- 1 teaspoon fresh lemon juice

DIRECTIONS

1. Melt some butter and sauté the onion for about 6–8 minutes.
2. Add the cream cheese and cook for about 2 minutes or until it's melted completely.
3. Stir in the water and spinach and cook for about 4–5 minutes.
4. Stir in the salt, black pepper, and lemon juice, and remove from heat.
5. Serve immediately.

NUTRITIONS

- Calories: 214 kcal
- Fat: 9.5g
- Fiber: 2.3g
- Carbohydrates: 2.1g
- Protein: 4.2g

PREPARATION TIME
15'

COOK TIME
15'

SERVING
4

INGREDIENTS

Tempura zucchinis:
- 1 ½ cups (200 g) almond flour
- 2 tablespoon heavy cream
- 1 teaspoon salt
- 2 tablespoon olive oil + extra for frying
- 1 ¼ cups (300 ml) water
- ½ tablespoon sugar-free maple syrup
- 2 large zucchinis, cut into 1-inch thick strips

Cream cheese dip:
- 8 ounces cream cheese, room temperature
- ½ cup (113 g) sour cream
- 1 teaspoon taco seasoning
- 1 scallion, chopped
- 1 green chili, deseeded and minced

DIRECTIONS

Tempura zucchinis:
1. In a bowl, mix the almond flour, heavy cream, salt, peanut oil, water, and maple syrup.
2. Dredge the zucchini strips in the mixture until well-coated.
3. Heat about four tablespoons of olive oil in a nonstick skillet.
4. Working in batches, use tongs to remove the zucchinis (draining extra liquid) into the oil.
5. Fry per side for 1 to 2 minutes and remove the zucchinis onto a paper towel-lined plate to drain grease.

Enjoy the zucchinis.
6. Cream cheese dip:
7. In a bowl or container, add the cream cheese, taco seasoning, sour cream, scallion, and green chili and mix.
8. Serve the tempura zucchinis with the cream cheese dip.

NUTRITIONS

- Calories: 316 kcal
- Fat: 8.4g
- Fiber: 9.3g
- Carbohydrates: 4.1g
- Protein: 5.1g

21. BACON AND FETA SKEWERS

 **PREPARATION TIME**
15'

 **COOK TIME**
10'

 **SERVING**
4

INGREDIENTS

- 2 pounds feta cheese, cut into 8 cubes
- 8 bacon slices
- 4 bamboo skewers, soaked
- 1 zucchini, cut into 8 bite-size cubes
- Salt and black pepper to taste
- 3 tablespoon almond oil for brushing

DIRECTIONS

1. Wrap each feta cube with a bacon slice.
2. Thread one wrapped feta on a skewer, add a zucchini cube, then another wrapped feta, and another zucchini.
3. Repeat the threading process with the remaining skewers.
4. Preheat a grill pan to medium heat, generously brush with the avocado oil and grill the skewer on both sides for 3 to 4 minutes per side or until the set is golden brown and the bacon cooked.
5. Serve afterward with the tomato salsa.

NUTRITIONS

- Calories: 290 kcal
- Fat: 15.1g
- Fiber: 4.2g
- Carbohydrates: 4.1g
- Protein: 11.8g

22. LOW-CARB THAI PEANUT SAUCE

PREPARATION TIME

5'

COOK TIME

5'

SERVING

6

INGREDIENTS

- ½ cup peanut butter, crisp
- 3 tablespoon chicken soup, warm, carb 0
- 3 tablespoons soy sauce
- 3 tablespoons hot sauce
- 2 tablespoons lime juice
- ½ ounces raw ginger, grated
- ½ tablespoon garlic
- ¼ teaspoon molasses, no sulfur
- 4 pineapple water enhancers, 0 carbs
- 1 tablespoon monk fruit or stevia to taste
- 1 tablespoon sesame oil
- 1 teaspoon fish sauce (optional-if needed)

DIRECTIONS

1. Whisk all ingredients together until smooth.
2. Cover in a non-reactive (glass is best) bottle.
3. Leave at least overnight before using it, this helps the flavor to blend.
4. Store in a tightly covered refrigerator

NUTRITIONS

- Energy (calories): 117 kcal
- Protein: 2.67 g
- Fat: 7.71 g
- Carbohydrates: 9.63 g

23. SPICY LEMON HERB SAUCE

PREPARATION TIME
15'

COOK TIME
1'

SERVING
4

INGREDIENTS

- 1 shallot, peeled and coarsely chopped
- 1 piece of garlic, peeled and crushed
- 1 bunch of roughly chopped parsley
- 1 bunch of mint, roughly chopped
- 1 bunch of roughly chopped coriander
- 2 lemons, peeled, juice
- olive cup olive oil
- 1 teaspoon salt
- 2 teaspoon freshly ground black pepper
- 1 teaspoon red pepper flakes

DIRECTIONS

1. In a blender or food processor, mix the shallots, garlic, herbs, and lemon zest.
2. Add lemon juice and olive oil and mix until a smooth sauce is formed. Season with salt, pepper, and red pepper flakes
3. Transfer the sauce to a closed container and refrigerate until use. The sauce can be stored for up to one week.

NUTRITIONS

- Calories: 390 kcal
- Fat: 37g
- Carbs: 17g
- Protein: 4g
- Sugars: 4g

24. ALL-PURPOSE EASY MUSTARD KETO SALAD DRESSING

PREPARATION TIME
5'

COOK TIME
5'

SERVING
4

INGREDIENTS

- 1 cup olive oil
- ¾ cup apple cider vinegar
- ¼ cup gray pom pom or other prepared mustard
- 1 tablespoon soy sauce
- 1 tablespoon Splenda
- 4 pieces of garlic
- 1 teaspoon salt
- 1 teaspoon black pepper

DIRECTIONS

1. Put all the ingredients in a Vitamix or other strong blender and blend for 1 minute until well emulsified.
2. Store in the refrigerator for up to 1 month and shake before use.
3. Use it as a salad, grilled meat, dip, or steamed vegetables to taste the wonderful flavor. This dressing dissolves in vegetables and gives a wonderful finish.

NUTRITIONS

- Calories: 262 kcal
- Carbohydrates: 1g
- Fat: 28g
- Saturated Fat: 4g
- Sodium: 506mg
- Potassium: 37mg
- Vitamin C: 0.6mg
- Calcium: 9mg
- Iron: 0.3mg

25. KETO ICE CREAM SANDWICH CHAFFLE

PREPARATION TIME
5'

COOK TIME
5'

SERVING
2

INGREDIENTS

- 2 tablespoons cocoa
- 2 tablespoons Monk fruit Confectioner's
- 1 egg
- ¼ teaspoon baking powder
- 1 tablespoon Heavy Whipped Cream
- Add selected keto ice cream

DIRECTIONS

1. Whip the egg in a small bowl.
2. Add the rest of the ingredients and mix well until smooth and creamy.
3. Pour half of the batter into a mini waffle maker and cook until fully cooked for 2 ½ to 3 minutes.
4. Allow the ice cream to cool completely before it's placed in the freezer.
5. Freeze all the way to solid.
6. Serve and beat the hot weather!

NUTRITIONS

- Calories: 158 kcal
- Calories from Fat: 141g
- Fat: 15.7g
- Sodium: 209mg
- Potassium: 128mg
- Carbohydrates: 9.9g
- Fiber: 2.9g
- Sugar: 0.9g
- Protein: 11.5g
- Vitamin A: 345 IU
- Calcium: 175mg
- Iron: 1.8mg

26. PEPPERONI PIZZA CHAFFLE

PREPARATION TIME
5'

COOK TIME
10'

SERVING
2

INGREDIENTS

For chaffle:
- ½ cup mozzarella
- 1 grade A large egg
- 1 tablespoon almond flour
- 1 teaspoon oregano
- 1 teaspoon garlic powder
- 1 teaspoon baking powder
- 1 teaspoon red pepper flakes
- 6 pepperonis

For sauce:
- ½ tablespoon tomato paste
- 1 Olive oil light rain (to make the paste a little thinner)
- A pinch of oregano

DIRECTIONS

1. Mix the egg, almond flour, garlic powder, oregano, red pepper flakes, and baking powder together in a bowl.
2. Add the mozzarella cheese and coat with the mixture evenly.
3. Spray your waffle maker with oil (if necessary) and heat it up to its maximum setting.
4. Cook the waffle, check it every 5 minutes until it becomes golden and crunchy.
5. While it's cooking the chaffle, to make the sauce, mix the tomato paste, olive oil, and oregano. If your sauce is too thick, it will be helped by a teaspoon of water.
6. Cut the chaffle and apply the sauce to the tomato.
7. Sprinkle on top with mozzarella cheese and top with pepperonis.
8. Microwave to melt the cheese and cook the pepperonis for 30 seconds
9. Serve and enjoy.

NUTRITIONS

- Calories: 258 kcal
- Calories from Fat: 141g
- Fat: 15.7g
- Sodium: 209mg
- Potassium: 128mg
- Carbohydrates: 9.9g
- Fiber: 2.9g
- Sugar: 0.9g
- Protein: 11.5g
- Vitamin A: 345 IU
- Calcium: 175mg
- Iron: 1.8mg

27. KETO CORNBREAD CHAFFLE

PREPARATION TIME
5'

COOK TIME
5'

SERVING
2

INGREDIENTS

- 1 egg
- ½ cup shredded cheddar cheese (or mozzarella cheese)
- 5 slice Jalapeno option-freshly picked or fresh
- 1 teaspoon of Frank's Red Hot Sauce
- ¼ teaspoon corn extract, is an essential secret ingredient
- Pinch of salt

DIRECTIONS

1. Preheat the mini waffle maker and place the eggs in a small bowl.
2. The remaining ingredients are added and combined until well absorbed.
3. Apply 1 tablespoon of shredded cheese to the waffle maker for 30 seconds before removing the mixture. It produces a very clean and friendly crust.
4. To a preheated waffle maker, add half of the mixture.
5. Cook for a total of 3-4 minutes. The more you cook it for the crunchier it gets.
6. Serve warm and enjoy.

NUTRITIONS

- Calories: 150 kcal
- Total Fat: 11.8g
- Cholesterol: 121mg
- Sodium: 1399.4mg
- Total Carbohydrate: 1.1g
- Dietary Fiber: 0g
- Sugars: 0.2g
- Protein: 9.6g
- Vitamin A: 134.1µg
- Vitamin C: 0.1mg T

28. LOW-CARB MINI PIZZA CHAFFLE

 **PREPARATION TIME** 5'

 **COOK TIME** 5'

 **SERVING** 2

INGREDIENTS

- 1 egg
- ½ cup mozzarella cheese shredded
- ¼ teaspoon of garlic powder
- ½ teaspoon Italian seasoning
- Salt and pepper

Toppings:
- Tomato sauce, cheese, pepperoni, etc.

DIRECTIONS

1. Put all ingredients in a bowl. Mix well.
2. Preheat the waffle maker. When it's hot, spray olive oil and put half of the dough in a mini waffle maker or put all of the dough in a large waffle maker. Cook each chaffle for 2-4 minutes.
3. Add the toppings and bake or fry the mini pizza until the cheese topping has melted.
4. Serve and enjoy!

NUTRITIONS

- Calories: 118 kcal
- Calories from Fat: 72g
- Fat: 8g
- Sodium: 207mg
- Potassium: 52mg
- Carbohydrates: 1g
- Fiber: 0.5g
- Sugar: 1g
- Protein: 9g
- Vitamin A: 308IU
- Calcium: 162mg
- Iron: 1mg

29. KETO CHAFFLE TACOS

PREPARATION TIME
5'

COOK TIME
5'

SERVING
2

INGREDIENTS

- ½ cup cheese cheddar or mozzarella cheese, shredded
- 1 egg
- ¼ teaspoon Italian seasoning
- 1 pound ground beef octopus seasoning ingredients
- 1 teaspoon chili powder
- 1 teaspoon cumin
- ½ teaspoon garlic powder
- ½ teaspoon cocoa powder
- ¼ teaspoon onion powder
- ¼ teaspoon salt
- 1/12 teaspoon smoked paprika

Taco meat seasoning for large lots

- ¼ cup chili powder
- ¼ cup grand cumin
- 2 tablespoons garlic powder
- 2 tablespoons cocoa powder
- 1 tablespoon onion powder
- 1 tablespoon
- 1 teaspoon smoked paprika

DIRECTIONS

1. Cook the minced meat first.
2. Add all taco meat seasonings. Cocoa powder is optional, but completely enhances the flavor of all the other seasonings.
3. While making the octopus meat, start making the keto chaffle.
4. Preheat the waffle maker. I am using a mini waffle maker.
5. First, whip the eggs in a small bowl.
6. Add shredded cheese and seasonings.
7. Put half of the chaffle mixture into a mini waffle maker and cook for about 3-4 minutes.
8. Cook the second half of the mixture repeatedly to make a second chaffle.
9. Add warm taco meat to the octopus chaffle.
10. Top it with lettuce, tomato, and cheese, and serve warm!

NUTRITIONS

- Calories: 118 kcal
- Calories from Fat: 141g
- Fat: 15.7g
- Sodium: 209mg
- Potassium: 128mg
- Carbohydrate: 9.9g
- Fiber: 2.9g
- Sugar: 0.9g
- Protein: 11.5g
- Vitamin A: 345 IU
- Calcium: 175mg
- Iron: 1.8mg

PREPARATION TIME
10'

COOK TIME
10'

SERVING
6

INGREDIENTS

- 500 g bovine bones (definitely also marrow bones)
- Liters of water
- 1 tablespoon of apple cider vinegar (optional)
- 1 pinch sea salt (optional)
- 1 bunch of soup vegetables
- 1 carrot
- 1 garlic clove
- 1 fresh onion
- 1 piece of ginger
- 1 teaspoon nutmeg (optional)

DIRECTIONS

1. Peel the carrot and onions and cut them into chunks. Wash the soup vegetables (celeriac, leeks, parsley) and cut into coarse pieces. Peel garlic and crush. Peel ginger and cut roughly.
2. Place the bones in a large saucepan and fry without fat.
3. Add the pre-cut vegetables to the bones and continue to roast together.
4. Fill the bones and vegetables with filtered water until everything is covered. Add 1 tablespoon of apple cider vinegar and parsley and bring to a boil.
5. Simmer for 3-4 hours. After 2-3 hours, if necessary, remove the marrow from the bones (continue to use) and continue to boil.
6. Bone broth through a sieve into another pot, season with coarse sea salt and other spices.
7. Divided it and freeze it or serve immediately:

NUTRITIONS

- Calories: 41 kcal
- Total Fat: 0.3g
- Cholesterol: 2.5mg
- Sodium: 486mg
- Potassium 24mg
- Total Carbohydrates: 0.6g
- Sugars: 0.5g
- Protein: 9.4g
- Vitamin A
- Vitamin C
- Calcium

31. KETO CHAFFLE STUFFING

PREPARATION TIME	COOK TIME	SERVING
20'	40'	4

INGREDIENTS

Basic chaffle ingredients
- ½ cup cheese mozzarella, cheddar cheese, or a combination of both
- 2 eggs
- ¼ teaspoon of garlic powder
- ½ teaspoon onion powder
- ½ teaspoon dried chicken seasoning
- ¼ teaspoon salt
- ¼ teaspoon pepper

Ingredients for filling
- 1 diced onion
- 2 celery stems
- 4 ounces mushrooms diced
- 4 cups butter for sautéing
- 3 eggs

DIRECTIONS

1. First, make a chaffle. This recipe makes four mini-chaffle.
2. Preheat mini waffle iron.
3. Preheat the oven to 350°F.
4. In a medium bowl, mix the chaffle ingredients.
5. Pour ¼ of the mixture into a mini waffle maker and cook each chaffle for about 4 minutes each.
6. When they are all cooked, set aside.
7. In a small skillet, fry the onions, celery, and mushrooms until soft.
8. In a separate bowl, split the chaffle into small pieces and add sautéed vegetables and three eggs. Mix until the ingredients are completely blended.
9. Add the mixture of fillings to a small casserole dish (about 4x4) and bake at 350°F for about 30-40 minutes.

NUTRITIONS

- Calories: 229 kcal
- Total Fat: 17.6g
- Cholesterol: 265.6mg
- Sodium: 350mg
- Total Carbohydrate: 4.6g
- Dietary Fiber: 1.1g
- Sugars: 2g
- Protein: 13.7g
- Vitamin A: 217.2 µg
- Vitamin C: 2.4mg

32. KETO CHAFFLE BREAKFAST SANDWICH

PREPARATION TIME
10'

COOK TIME
10'

SERVING
6

INGREDIENTS

- Two large eggs, split
- ½ cup minced mozzarella or hard cheese
- ¼ cup almond flour (optional)
- 2 slice bacon (60 g/2.1 ounces)
- 1 slice of tomato (27 g/1 ounce)
- Sliced cheese such as cheddar cheese (28 g/1 ounce)

DIRECTIONS

1. Preheat the mini waffle iron. Whisk one of the eggs in a small bowl. If necessary, add almond flour and mix well. If only eggs are used, the dough will be very smooth.
2. Sprinkle a quarter of the minced mozzarella cheese (about ½ ounces/14 g) on a waffle iron and sprinkle half of the whipped egg on top. Alternatively, whisk eggs directly with mozzarella cheese.
3. Sprinkle a quarter more of mozzarella (about ½ ounces/14 g) and close the iron. Cook for 2-3 minutes until the waffles come off easily. Repeat for the second waffle.

Keto chaffle breakfast sandwich

4. Cook the bacon slices in a small skillet and scramble the remaining eggs in the same skillet.
5. Put on top of the waffles some sliced cheese, tomatoes, bacon, and eggs, finish with another waffle on top and serve.

NUTRITIONS

- Energy (calories): 58 kcal
- Protein: 4.55 g
- Fat: 4.19 g
- Carbohydrates: 0.61 g

33. KETO PIZZA CHAFFLE

PREPARATION TIME
10'

COOK TIME
7'

SERVING
6

INGREDIENTS

- 1 egg
- ½ cup mozzarella cheese shredded
- Just a pinch of Italian seasoning
- Pizza sauce
- 1 tablespoon sugar
- Top with shredded cheese or pepperoni (or favorite topping)

DIRECTIONS

1. Preheat the Dash waffle maker.
2. Whip the egg and the seasonings together in a small bowl.
3. Mix with the shredded cheese.
4. Add a teaspoon of shredded cheese to the preheated waffle maker and cook for about 30 seconds. This is going to help develop a more crisp crust.
5. Add half the mixture to the waffle maker and cook for about 4 minutes until golden brown and slightly crispy.
6. Cut the waffle and add the remaining mixture to the waffle maker to make the second waffle.
7. Top with a spoonful of pizza sauce, shredded cheese, and pepperoni. Microwave it for about 20 seconds and serve.

NUTRITIONS

- Calories: 258 kcal
- Calories from Fat: 141g
- Fat: 15.7g
- Sodium: 209mg
- Potassium: 128mg
- Carbohydrates: 9.9g
- Fiber: 2.9g
- Sugar: 0.9g
- Protein: 11.5g
- Vitamin A: 345 IU
- Calcium: 175mg

34. AVOCADO EGG SALAD

PREPARATION TIME
10'

COOK TIME
5'

SERVING
6

INGREDIENTS

- 4 hard-boiled eggs
- 2 avocados
- 30 g Greek yogurt
- ½ lime, juiced
- 1 teaspoon granular mustard
- 1-2 spring onions(in fine rings)
- Pepper
- Salt

DIRECTIONS

1. The preparation is so simple that it actually requires no instructions. When all the ingredients are prepared this salad is ready in less than 5 minutes.
2. Peel and dice the hard-boiled eggs.
3. When choosing the avocados, you should take ripe ones, which are already a bit soft, because they will be crushed later anyway. Cut the avocados into two equal halves while you remove the core and scrape them out with a tablespoon.
4. Then add the avocado with the mustard, the yogurt, and the lime juice to a bowl and crush everything into a fine puree. Then add the cubed eggs and half of the spring onions, mix and season with salt and pepper to taste.

NUTRITIONS

- Calories: 119.0 kcal
- Total Fat: 8.7g
- Saturated Fat: 1.8g
- Polyunsaturated Fat: 1.4g
- Monounsaturated Fat: 4.3g
- Cholesterol: 124.8mg
- Sodium: 192.9mg
- Potassium: 190.5mg
- Total Carbohydrate: 3.4g
- Dietary Fiber: 2.0g
- Sugars: 0.8g
- Protein: 7.2g

35. KETO SAUSAGE BALL CHAFFLE

PREPARATION TIME
5'

COOK TIME
3'

SERVING
2

INGREDIENTS

- 1 pound bulk Italian sausage
- 1 cup almond flour
- 2 teaspoons baking powder
- 1 cup shredded cheddar cheese
- ¼ cup grated parmesan cheese
- 1 egg, or if you are allergic to eggs, you can use flax eggs

DIRECTIONS

1. Heat the maker of mini waffles to average.
2. Put all the ingredients in a big bowl and combine well by hand.
3. Place a paper plate to catch any drops under the waffle maker.
4. In a hot waffle maker, spoon a 3 tablespoon of the mixture.
5. Cook for a total of 3 minutes. Switch over and cook for another 2 minutes to get a crisp look.

NUTRITIONS

- Calories: 302 kcal
- Calories from Fat: 141g
- Fat: 15.7g
- Sodium: 209mg
- Potassium: 128mg
- Carbohydrates: 9.9g
- Fiber: 2.9g
- Sugar: 0.9g
- Protein: 11.5g
- Vitamin A: 345 IU
- Calcium: 175mg
- Iron: 1.8mg

36. KETO BLUEBERRY CHAFFLE

 **PREPARATION TIME** 5'

 **COOK TIME** 15'

 **SERVING** 5

INGREDIENTS

- 1 cup mozzarella cheese
- 2 tablespoons almond flour
- 1 teaspoon baking powder
- 2 eggs
- 1 teaspoon cinnamon
- 2 teaspoon sweetener
- 3 tablespoons and ¼ cup blueberry, separated

DIRECTIONS

1. Heat up your mini waffle maker.
2. Place the mozzarella cheese, almond flour, baking powder, milk, cinnamon, and blueberries in a mixing bowl. Mix well in order to blend all the ingredients together.
3. Spray the nonstick cooking spray on your mini waffle maker.
4. Add in a little bit less than ¼ cup of blueberry keto waffle batter.
5. Close the lid and cook for 3-5 minutes of the chaffle. Check to see if it's crispy and golden at the 3-minute mark. If it is not or if it sticks to the top of the waffle cooker, close the lid and cook for 1-2 more minutes.
6. Serve with a drop of swerve sweetener or keto syrup.

NUTRITIONS

- Calories: 116 kcal
- Carbohydrates: 3g
- Protein: 8g
- Fat: 8g
- Saturated Fat: 4g
- Cholesterol: 83mg
- Sodium: 166mg
- Potassium: 142mg
- Fiber: 1g
- Vitamin C: 1mg
- Calcium: 177mg
- Iron: 1mg

37. KETO CHOCOLATE TWINKIE COPYCAT CHAFFLE

PREPARATION TIME
5'

COOK TIME
12'

SERVING
3

INGREDIENTS

- 2 tablespoons of butter, cooled
- 2 ounces cream cheese, softened
- 2 large eggs, room temperature
- 1 teaspoon of vanilla essence
- ¼ cup Locanto confectionery
- Pinch of pink salt
- ¼ cup almond flour
- 2 tablespoons coconut powder
- 2 tablespoons cocoa powder
- 1 teaspoon baking powder

DIRECTIONS

1. Preheat the Corndog Maker.
2. Melt the butter and let it cool for a minute.
3. In the butter, whisk the eggs until smooth.
4. Add the cinnamon, vanilla, sweetener and blend well.
5. Add the almond flour, coconut flour, cacao powder, and baking powder. Mix until well blended.
6. Fill each well with 2 tablespoons of batter and spread evenly.
7. Close the lid and let it cook for 4 minutes.
8. Remove and cool it down.

NUTRITIONS

- Calories: 104 kcal
- Total Fat: 6.2g
- Cholesterol: 67.1mg
- Sodium: 485.5mg
- Total Carbohydrate: 5.3g
- Dietary Fiber: 1.7g
- Sugars: 1.6g
- Protein: 4.4g
- Vitamin A: 80.1µg
- Vitamin C: 0mg

38. LOW-CARB BBQ SAUCE

 **PREPARATION TIME**
5'

 **COOK TIME**
15'

 **SERVING**
1

INGREDIENTS

- ¼ cup Sukrin Gold brown sugar, or your favorite sweetener
- ¼ cup apple cider vinegar
- ¼ cup white vinegar
- ½ cup of water
- 2 tablespoons eal butter
- 1 (6 ounces) can of tomato paste
- 1 teaspoon garlic powder
- 1 teaspoon onion powder
- 1 teaspoon dried yellow mustard
- 1 teaspoon salt
- 1 teaspoon cayenne pepper, optional
- 1 teaspoon liquid smoke, optional

DIRECTIONS

1. If you like a thinner sauce, add more water until you have reached the desired thickness.
2. If you like a sauce that is sourer, add a little more vinegar.
3. The liquid smoke is easy to use; a little goes a long way!
4. This recipe can be adapted very easily to different sweeteners. Using a white sweetener will lead to a more red-colored sauce.
5. The butter makes a beautiful glossy finish and helps the sauce to adhere to anything you brush on.
6. Store in the refrigerator for up to 2 weeks.

NUTRITIONS

- Calories: 18 kcal
- Total Fat: 1g
- Saturated Fat: 0g
- Trans Fat: 0g
- Unsaturated Fat: 0g
- Carbohydrates: 2g
- Fiber: 0g
- Sugar alcohols: 0g
- Protein: 0g

39. PESTO ZOODLES

PREPARATION TIME
15'

COOK TIME
10'

SERVING
4

INGREDIENTS

Pesto:
- 2 cups fresh basil leaves
- 1 piece crushed garlic
- ⅓ cup pine nuts
- 3 tablespoons grated parmesan cheese
- 1 cup extra virgin olive oil, or as required
- Freshly ground black pepper with salt

Zoodles:
- 1 tablespoon extra virgin olive oil
- 1 onion, sliced
- 4 zucchini, cut into noodles
- Parmesan curls needed for garnish
- Red pepper flakes required for garnish (optional)

DIRECTIONS

1. To make the pesto: add the basil, garlic, pine nuts, and parmesan cheese in a food processor or mixer until it is chopped vigorously.
2. With the food processor running, slowly add the olive oil and mix until the pesto becomes a thick paste. To adjust consistency, add olive oil as needed. Season with salt and pepper.
3. To make the zoodles: heat the oil on medium heat with a broad frying pan. Add the onions and fry for 4-5 minutes before softening. Serve with zucchini noodles and fry for 4-5 minutes before becoming soft.
4. Remove the pesto and mix until well coated with noodles.
5. Serve with warm parmesan curls and red pepper flakes.

NUTRITIONS

- Calories: 281 kcal
- Fat: 29g
- Carbs: 2g
- Protein: 6g
- Sugars: 1g

Zoodles:
- Calories: 89 kcal
- Fat: 4g
- Carbs: 12g
- Protein: 3g
- Sugars: 9g

40. RICE BREAD WITH SOY SAUCE

PREPARATION TIME
3 1/2 HOURS

COOK TIME
20'

SERVING
8

INGREDIENTS

- 4 ½ cups almond flour
- 1 cup, rice, cooked
- 1 egg
- 2 tablespoons soy sauce
- 2 teaspoons dried yeast
- 2 tablespoons melted butter
- 1 tablespoon brown sugar
- 2 teaspoons salt

DIRECTIONS

1. Pour 1 ¼ cups of water, and soy sauce; add the egg.
2. Put in the flour and rice.
3. Put ghee, sugar, and salt in different corners of the mold. Make a groove in the flour, and put in the yeast.
4. Bake in "normal, medium crust" mode for about 20 minutes at 200 F.
5. Bread is ready to eat when cooled.

NUTRITIONS

- Carbohydrates 3.6 g
- Fats 4.2 g
- Protein 9.1 g
- Calories 321

41. BREAD WITH TURKEY AND RAISINS COPYCAT CHAFFLE

PREPARATION TIME
3 HOURS

COOK TIME
20'

SERVING
8

INGREDIENTS

- 20 oz. turkey
- 1 cup of raisins
- 2 big onions
- 2 cloves chopped garlic
- 1 cup of milk
- 25 oz. almond flour
- 10 oz. rye flour
- 3 teaspoons dry yeast
- 1 egg
- 3 tablespoons sunflower oil
- 1 teaspoon sugar
- Himalayan salt

DIRECTIONS

1. Soak the raisins in the warm water for 10 minutes.
2. Boil the turkey meat with the salt on medium heat until soft. You can use the turkey breast or fillet.
3. Blend the cooked and soft turkey meat using a food processor until it has a smooth consistency.
4. Chop the onions and garlic and then fry them until clear and caramelized.
5. Combine the yeast with the warm water, mixing until smooth consistency.
6. Combine all the ingredients with the yeast, turkey, onions, raisins, garlic and then mix and knead well.
7. Pour some oil into a bread machine and place the dough into the bread maker. Cover the dough with the towel and leave for 1 hour.
8. Close the lid and turn the bread machine on the basic program.
9. Bake the bread until the medium crust for 20 minutes at 300 F and after the bread is ready take it out and leave for 1 hour covered with the towel and only then you can slice the bread.

NUTRITIONS

- Carbohydrates 4.9 g
- Fats 6.8 g
- Protein 34 g
- Calories 329

42. BREAD WITH BEEF AND PEANUTS

PREPARATION TIME

3 HOURS

COOK TIME

20'

SERVING

8

INGREDIENTS

- 15 oz. beef meat
- 5 oz. Herbes de Provence
- 2 big onions
- 2 cloves chopped garlic
- 1 cup of milk
- 20 oz. almond flour
- 10 oz. rye flour
- 3 teaspoons dry yeast
- 1 egg
- 3 tablespoons sunflower oil
- 1 tablespoon sugar
- Sea salt
- ground black pepper
- red pepper

DIRECTIONS

1. Sprinkle the beef meat with the Herbes de Provence, salt, black, and red pepper and marinate in bear for overnight.
2. Cube the beef and fry in a skillet or a wok on medium heat until soft (for around 20 minutes).
3. Chop the onions and garlic and then fry them until clear and caramelized.
4. Combine all the ingredients except for the beef and then mix well.
5. Combine the beef pieces and the dough and mix in the bread machine.
6. Close the lid and turn the bread machine on the basic program.
7. Bake the bread until the medium crust and after the bread is ready take it out and leave for 1 hour covered with the towel and only then you can slice the bread.

NUTRITIONS

- Carbohydrates 4 g
- Fats 42 g
- Protein 27 g
- Calories 369

CONCLUSION

Thank you for making it through the end. Taking your first steps towards a healthy life is probably one of the hardest and bravest things a person can do. By choosing to follow a ketogenic diet, you are taking that challenging first step. Use the information you have learned throughout this book to help make this transition easier and more fulfilling. Just know that it doesn't matter how old you are, how big you are, or how physically active you are, because all of that can be changed through taking that first step. The best place to start off would be to figure out your numbers and then go through your house and start trashing the foods you will no longer have.

This is going to test you, and it won't be easy, but once you start seeing the results, it will be fulfilling. You will notice some quick changes, and while those may slow down over time, if you stick to the diet, you will see the weight fall off. It's easy to enjoy this diet, as well. The important thing is to get creative, and you will soon find that you can enjoy any meal you enjoyed before, but with a carb-friendly twist.

Ensure that you have your goals set and have all of the food that you will need to be successful before you start. Make sure you have lots of healthy fats because these are what will keep you full from now on. You can also play around with your macros to find that sweet spot that works well for you. The important thing is that you make this diet work for you. Now, go get started.

The first thing you have to do is write down the motivation or reasons why you want to change. This change must end at a goal. Wanting to lose weight isn't good enough. You need to be motivated due to the consequence of being overweight. Again losing weight isn't a clear goal. You need to set a certain weight you want to get to. You need to write it down legibly along with your reason. For example, "I will lose 50 pounds to help prevent me from getting diabetes." This is a great goal. Self-control and willpower can't happen until these other steps happen. Writing a goal along with two specifics and reading that goal every day will create a trigger by giving the goal specifics.

The next thing you need to do is monitor how you act toward the goal. When trying to lose weight, you need to keep a diet journal. You will need to write down every single thing you drink and eat. Each evening writes out your plans for the next day's meals. That evening, you will audit yourself for either your failures or successes by writing on the same page what you really did drink and eat. Keep doing this every evening. You have to be honest with yourself about why you either failed or succeeded. This last part is what is very powerful. It is called self-introspection. This is the key that lets you see your habits. You will be able to make changes and get rid of any bad habits you see. This helps you strengthen your willpower and form good habits.

As with anything in life, there are going to be some downsides. This goes for the keto diet, too, but it isn't dangerous. Many bad things such as kidney stones, gastrointestinal distress, decreased bone density, high cholesterol, mineral and vitamin deficiencies, and increased risk of heart disease can be reduced by drinking more water and taking supplements

As long as you make sure you are getting lots of electrolytes and water, you shouldn't have a problem.